EAT BACON, DON'T JOG

Thanks!
Grant Petersen

EAT BACON, DON'T JOG

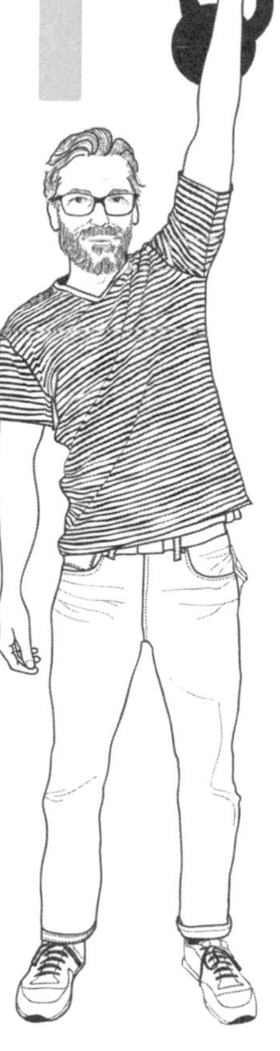

Get Strong. Get Lean. No Bullshit.

GRANT PETERSEN

Illustrations by Amanda Sim

WORKMAN PUBLISHING
NEW YORK

Disclaimer: The author is not a doctor or a health field professional. The knowledge shared in the book is from his general education in the subject, as well as his experience. Before beginning any change in your health regimen, consult a professional health care practitioner. Neither the author nor the publisher shall be liable or responsible for any loss, injury, or damage allegedly arising from any information or suggestions contained in this book.

Published simultaneously in Canada by Thomas Allen & Son Limited.

Library of Congress Cataloging-in-Publication Data is available.

ISBN 978-0-7611-8054-8

Design by Jean-Marc Troadec

Workman books are available at special discounts when purchased in bulk for premiums and sales promotions as well as for fund-raising or educational use. Special editions or book excerpts can also be created to specification. For details, contact the Special Sales Director at the address below, or send an email to specialmarkets@workman.com.

Workman Publishing Company, Inc.
225 Varick Street
New York, NY 10014-4381
workman.com

WORKMAN is a registered trademark of Workman Publishing Co., Inc.

Printed in the United States of America
First printing November 2014

10 9 8 7 6 5 4 3 2 1

DEDICATION

As always, to Mary, Kate, and Anna, and to my incredibly generous boss and coworkers at RBW, all of whom cut me slack in the writing of this book and guinea-pigged many of the recipes as a backup for my own too-tolerant palate.

ACKNOWLEDGMENTS

All of the people I've learned this stuff from, many of whom are named in the last chapter.

The people at Workman Publishing, in particular Suzie Bolotin, David Schiller, Beth Levy, Selina Meere, Jessica Wiener, and Jenny Mandel, with extra thanks to Mary Ellen O'Neill, who saves me from myself and makes me sound better than I am.

Amanda Sim, for her patience and fine illustrations.

Vassily Filipov, the strongest person I know and the most knowledgeable about muscles and exercise.

Ken Ford, who navigated me through the sharky waters of the science entries. If I left out an enzyme or critical fluid along the way, it's my fault.

John Gallagher, who rescued me from an ocean of authoritative yet conflicting information on the damnable Internet related to camel guts, horse guts, and rabbit guts. You can take what you're about to read to the bank.

Danielle Svetcov, for always coming through. Thanks, Svetcov!

CONTENTS

Introduction xiii

Food basics

01 It comes down to insulin, but it starts with carbohydrates . . 2
02 Carbohydrate primer, and why it's OK to eat less kale 4
03 How to stop being so hungry all day long, day after day 6
04 Fasting made easy 7
05 Moderation is not one-size-fits-all 9
06 Variety is overrated 10
07 You eat less often when you eat more fat and fewer carbs . . . 12
08 The dangers of eating too few carbs 13
09 Too much protein makes you fatter, not stronger 14
10 Get most of your calories from fat 15
11 How to eat a sandwich 16
12 Get off your lite version of the sumo wrestler weight-gain program 17
13 Four low-carb diets 19
14 You need food, not a pyramid or a plate 22
15 The most important meal of the day . . . to skip 24
16 Ten dinners, minimal carbs 25

Food particulars

17 The good fats 28

18 The bad fats 30

19 Keep your fats cool, or at least don't let them smoke 32

20 Drink a fatty breakfast 34

21 The whole grains ruse 35

22 All corn is candy corn 38

23 The fruit ruse 40

24 In vegetables, darker is bitterer is better 41

25 Never order an egg white omelet 43

26 Crack your own nuts 44

27 Olive oil is good, but not God 46

28 God is a coconut 47

29 How to get a figure like a potato 49

30 Salt and blood pressure, simplified 51

31 Soybeans: The honeymoon is over; the nutrition is overrated 53

32 Greek yogurt or none at all 54

33 Booze trumps junk 55

34 Going low-carb without going no-chocolate 57

35 Quickie guide to fake sugars (which are not really fake) ... 58

36 Eight foods to avoid at all costs 59

37 Eleven foods to eat with gusto 61

38 If you can afford this book, you can afford good food 64

39 Viva canned fish! 66

Exercise basics

40 Don't jog . . . 68

41 What kind of exercise works best? . . . 70

42 If your workout requires special clothing, it's the wrong kind of workout . . . 71

43 If you eat sugar, you can't exercise off your fat. . . . 72

44 When you're a fat-burner, you *will* exercise off fat . . . 74

45 If you can't jog yourself skinny, why are the world's best distance runners skinny? . . . 75

46 When the goal is strength, high reps waste time . . . 76

47 Write your routine on a 3-by-5-inch card, then follow it . . . 77

48 Make the most of a gym . . . 78

49 Mixing work and play wrecks both . . . 80

50 Don't cheat your muscles with momentum . . . 81

51 Walking is a big part of the plan . . . 82

52 Sit down at work or at home, but not both . . . 83

53 Stretch dynamically, not statically . . . 84

54 Don't make a big production of warming down . . . 86

Exercise particulars

55 Russian push-ups . . . 88

56 Janda sit-ups . . . 90

57 Push-ups with benches, chairs, and balls . . . 93

58 Pull up like a monkey . . . 94

59 Dips . . . 96

60 Crawl like a bug, but less efficiently . . . 98

61 Squat right 100
62 Jump like a kangaroo 102
63 The amazing kettlebell 103
64 Kettlebell two-hand swing 105
65 Kettlebell squat 109
66 Kettlebell snatch 110
67 Kettlebell Turkish get-up 113
68 Kettlebell clean, squat, press 116
69 Windmills, with and without a kettlebell 120
70 The brutal Tabata 123
71 Killer burpees 125
72 Countdowns 128
73 Repetitive countdowns 129
74 Fibonacci 130
75 Using the potentially deadly ab wheel 132
76 Medicine ball fetch 134
77 Sprint without pulling up lame 136
78 Any hill in your neighborhood is like a free public gym 138
79 Turning your bicycle into exercise gear 139
80 Hotel exercising 140
81 On tired or lazy days, spread it out 141

What's going on inside?

82 Ape + fish and fat + 2.8 million years = you 144
83 After millions of years of eating meat, your digestive system has grown to prefer it 148
84 When picking a food, go by your guts 149

85 Feed your guts, too 154

86 You're technically an omnivore, but your digestive system is 98 percent carnivore. 156

87 Hunger and homeostasis 157

88 Running more on ketones, less on glucose 159

89 Cancer thrives on glucose but can't live on ketones 162

90 How to make more fat and how to burn it up 163

91 Cholesterol, triglycerides, and artery health. 164

92 Diabetes primer for nondiabetics 165

93 Understand and test your own blood sugar. 166

94 In for a penny, in for a pound: Test your ketones, too . . . 168

95 Is your spit making you fat? 171

96 Alzheimer's: diabetes of the brain? 173

97 A survey isn't a study, a correlation isn't a cause, and an observation is just somebody looking at something . . 175

What to think about now

98 You can be fat and happy, but can you be fat and healthy? . . 178

99 If your child is overweight 179

100 Have you ever followed bad advice? 180

101 Pros and cons of being a teenage eater 181

102 Recalibrate your taste buds 182

103 Cats and dogs are carnivores, so feed them carne. 183

104 Bad advice from the pros 184

105 When animals are available, eat them 186

106 Don't let the clock be the boss of your piehole 187

Recipes

FANTASTIC FAKE PANCAKES 190

FAKE PIZZA WITH NO CRUST 191

FANTASTIC FAKE QUICHE 192

GREEN SOUP 193

REAL RATATOUILLE 195

DIABETES-SAFE CROUTONS 197

SUPER WHITE "CEREAL" 198

FUN WITH CREAM 199

CHOCKOROONS 200

COCONUT BUTTER 201

BLUE CHEESE AND CHERRY TOMATO SOUP ... 202

FANTASTIC BLUE CHEESE DRESSING 203

JAPANEASY SOUP 204

BLUE CHEESE AND MACADAMIA NUT DESSERT 205

BREAKFAST CHOCOLATE 206

Outgrow this book 209

BOOKS 210

WEBSITES AND BLOGS 216

INDEX 217

INTRODUCTION

Eat Bacon, Don't Jog will derail your thinking on food and workouts. In it, I'll explain why your attempts to lose weight permanently have failed, and how eating nutritious fat and enduring short bursts of intense exercise will reverse that. You'll be able to make sense of past failures and will gain raging confidence that the program you're about to start will work.

In the mid- to late 1990s, when I was in my forties, I noticed that three decades of what seemed to be a perfect diet and exercise program wasn't working. For thirty years I'd avoided junk food, eating mostly oat bran, whole grains, egg whites, lean meat, fresh fruit, nonfat dairy, salads with no dressing. For thirty years I beat myself up and got all sweaty for one to three hours a day. I rode my bike hard every day, wore out a NordicTrack, and got frustrated on a rowing machine because I couldn't get my heart rate high enough. And I was still gaining weight. I wasn't fat by American standards, but I wasn't as lean as I should have been with all that "ideal" food and obsessive cardio. It got to the point that I was exercising just to avoid gaining weight faster, and no matter what, I was always the hungriest person within a hundred yards.

I was obsessed with being healthy because both my great-grandfather and grandfather died from heart attacks at age forty-seven. My dad made it to seventy-seven, but I figured genetics were against me. I was eating about 3,200 calories a day and burning up about half that in exercise. I knew a pound of fat has 3,500 calories and I understood the math of weight gain and loss, so I saw no way to get off the treadmill. Exercise that used to be play turned into work. I believed, as so many people do, that it is possible to exercise more and eat less and keep it up for a lifetime. That's the conventional wisdom, and it's the biggest lie in health.

As the disclaimer a few pages back highlights, I am not a doctor. But let me ask you this: How helpful has your doctor been? Not a lot, I'm guessing, or you wouldn't be holding this book. In any case, in the section Outgrow This Book, I list more authoritative sources for much of the same information I cover in *Eat Bacon, Don't Jog*. Read them for more of the science behind it all, and then find a doctor who knows about this science and will discuss it with you. Until then, you're best off eating lots of fat, a little protein, and some dark green leaves.

GRANT PETERSEN

FOOD BASICS

When you fail to lose weight, blame the diet. Really. A weight loss program that requires restraint, small portions, reduced calories, *and* more exercise is doomed from the start. It can work for a few miserable weeks, but it isn't sustainable, and when you fail you'll blame yourself. Then, after some time off from dieting and some weight gain, you try another diet with a different name that works in the same way and gives you the same results.

In the first two chapters, Food Basics and Food Particulars, I will explore three important points:

- Lowering your insulin is your salvation.
- Fat is your friend.
- Your excess body fat is due to the high-carb food you eat, not the calories you eat or exercise you avoid.

01 It comes down to insulin, but it starts with carbohydrates

When you eat cotton candy, bread, fruit, soda, or pasta, your body converts the carbs in them to a kind of sugar called glucose, and the glucose goes into your blood. I use the terms *sugar* and *glucose* interchangeably throughout the book. When you eat carbs, your blood glucose rises. Your blood sugar rises. It's the same thing.

When you eat carbs, your blood sugar rises. Your body treats glucose in your blood as poison, and your pancreas leaps to the rescue by secreting insulin, a hormone that determines where you get your energy from; what you burn for calories. When you eat carbs and raise your sugar, then your insulin, you burn sugar, not fat. You can think of this as your body's way of lowering the levels of poison glucose—burning it up.

So, yes—the insulin gets the glucose out of your blood—saving your life—and into your cells to be burned as energy so you can move, walk, run, ride a bike. And that's the last good thing insulin does.

THE INSULIN HIT LIST

- Insulin converts calories to fat. Even the calories from fat-free food become body fat.
- Insulin stores fat on your hips, belly, back—wherever you tend to pack it on, insulin puts it there.
- Insulin prevents you from using body fat as fuel. When you exercise hard and long, you think you're burning body fat, but you're not. Insulin won't let you burn off body fat.

- Insulin keeps you hungry. It makes you want more of the same carbohydrates that started the cycle in the first place.

And it doesn't stop there. Insulin is also a force behind many of the diseases we either live with or fear. Reducing insulin levels is *the* key to losing fat and *a* key to getting healthier, and there is only one way to do it: Quit eating carbohydrates. Not fat. Not protein. Carbohydrates.

Insulin is the problem. Eating carbohydrates drives up insulin. Cutting way back on carbs lowers your insulin levels, and that is the solution.

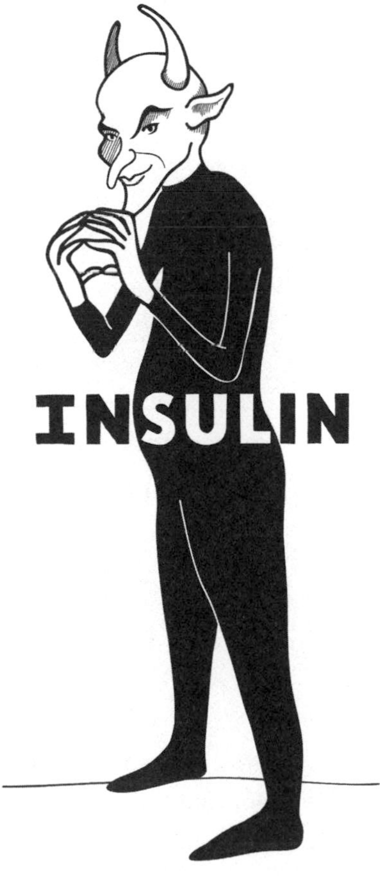

02 Carbohydrate primer, and why it's OK to eat less kale

Most carbohydrates are cheap and tasty, so we eat *a lot* of them. As munchies, as main meals, as quick pick-me-ups and energy boosts, as food mops for a sloppy plate, as holiday and special-occasion treats. We drink them as sodas, sports drinks, juice, and alcohol.

The worst carbohydrates are the pure sugars and syrups that come in candy and cookies and soda, and the refined carbohydrates (wheat without the bran or germ, for instance) used in white bread and fancy pastries. These simple carbs send your sugar and insulin levels skyrocketing, and they do it right after you have eaten them. If your body was burning fat before you ate them, eating them jacked up your insulin levels and put a halt to the fat burning.

The so-called good carbohydrates are natural, unprocessed ones like fruit, root vegetables, and whole grains. They're "complex" because the carbs are attached to plant fiber so it takes them longer to break down into glucose, so there's a smaller and delayed increase in blood sugar and insulin—compared to the carbs in a Coke.

But when the topic is weight gain, any carbohydrate breaks down to sugar and leads to high insulin levels and fat-making. It's easy to avoid the worst carbs, but the "good carbs" are even more dangerous because, like the enemy you don't recognize, they trick you. You gobble and guzzle them with abandon because they're natural and you've been told they're good for you. But here's the truth: the banana you eat with a glass of fresh-squeezed organic orange juice does more to keep you hungry and fat than the candy bar and Coke you don't go near. At least the candy and Coke make no pretense of being good for you.

The best carbs are the least harmful ones, and they are greens, especially leaves—kale, chard, cabbage, spinach, etc. It's not because of their nutrition, but because they have these three things in their favor:

- They're mostly water.
- They're low in sugar.
- What little sugar they have is bound up in cellulose, so it's not completely digestible.

Cellulose is the structural part of a plant. It makes celery sticklike and keeps chard from being totally floppy. Extracting all of the nutrients from the greens requires digesting the cellulose, but *that* requires cellulase, an enzyme we don't have (plant-eating herbivores do). The nutrients in the plant are also in the cellulose jail, so despite the high vitamin and mineral scores of kale, we don't access all of them. In a sense, eating nutrient-rich kale is like swallowing an undissolvable vitamin and mineral pill. When the nutrients are identified in a laboratory, the "digestion" of those nutrients is artificial and complete, but when you eat kale, your body says, *What are you doing, man? I can't digest this!*—and ejects it out your back door as fast as possible.

Eating refined carbohydrates, on the other hand, is like ingesting a carbohydrate capsule with a sugar coating that breaks down instantly and unleashes a torrent of sugar into a digestive system that responds to it by making you fat and sick and hungry.

03 How to stop being so hungry all day long, day after day

There are two ways to avoid that soul-crushing feeling of being hungry: eat until you have no more room and get fatter, or eat lots of fat and almost no carbohydrates and don't get fat.

When you limit your carbs to 50 grams or less a day—a slice of bread and a banana, for instance—and replace carbohydrates with good fat from animals, animal products, and selected plants (coconuts, macadamia nuts, avocados, and olives top the list), you'll get your calories from stored body fat, and that's what stops hunger. Even if you're relatively lean, you have plenty of body fat to supply your energy needs. Cut the carbs, eat more fat, and tame that raging appetite. That's how it works.

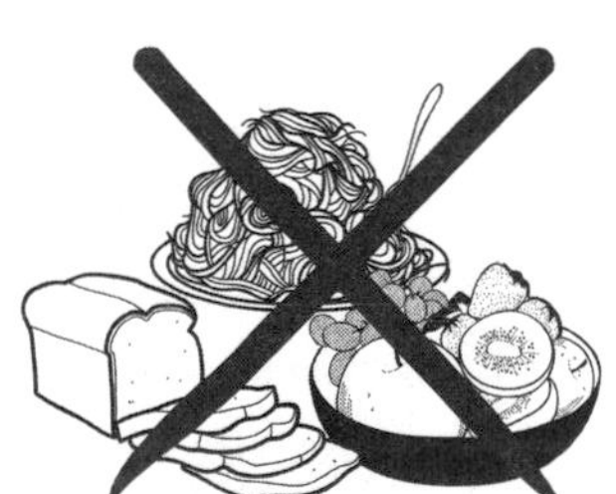

04 Fasting made easy

Whatever spiritual, bowel-cleansing, detoxifying, and generally suspect benefits the Eastern mystics and fasting fanatics may tout, the undeniable benefit of fasting is a lowering of blood sugar and a consequent lowering of blood insulin. When you cut out all food (including carbs), your blood-insulin level will drop, you'll start to burn body fat, and you'll stop being hungry. But starvation, even if only for a day, is a dreary and unnecessary way to get there. Besides, when you starve one day, it's easy to eat too much the next day. If you want to fast to reduce insulin, here are two ways that work just as well and don't make you miserable with cravings.

- The 18-hour fast: For a 24-hour period, clump all of your high-fat, low-carb eating into 6 hours. Pick any six-hour period: 8 to 2 o'clock, noon to 6, 6 to 12, or whatever you like. This approach wards off hunger while you fast the subsequent 18 hours. The 18 hours of fasting gives your body time to burn up whatever glucose is in your blood, which reduces your insulin and fat storage. This eating pattern is a perfectly healthy way to eat forever, although real life and social pressures (business lunches, for instance) may interfere.
- The all-day 90 percent fat fast: For 24 hours, eat nothing but cheese, homemade unsugared whipped cream, coconut oil, olive oil, butter, bacon, 2 to 4 ounces of fatty meat, or up to six eggs, depending on how big you are. Let the amount follow your hunger, but the point is to concentrate on eating or drinking fat. That's why it should be pork bacon,

not turkey bacon; and cream, not just whole milk. If you like Brie, get the triple-cream kind (or if you don't like Brie, try Cowgirl Creamery's Mt. Tam cheese).

On this nonfast fast you get to eat whenever you want. You won't be tempted to wash down a pound of bacon with a quart of cream, because without the insulin to make you ravenous you simply won't be hungry for that much food. When 90 percent of your calories come from fat and zero come from carbohydrates, your insulin plummets, just as it would in a water-only fast, but with less hunger.

Once you've done a few fat-only days, you'll find it easy to eat just one main, fatty meal a day. It may be a meaty, cheesy salad—not because the greens are necessary, but because they help fill up the vessel, add color, and help the meat last longer—like Hamburger Helper without the grains. Scatter a few fatty snacks like cheese or nuts throughout the day, and you'll lower your insulin, lose weight, and get healthier without the misery of starvation.

05 Moderation is not one-size-fits-all

It may feel like moderation when you cut your bread supply in half and limit yourself to a small pile of pasta. But the true gauge of moderation isn't your hunger; it's the glucose in your blood.

Some lucky people are insulin-sensitive, meaning that it takes just a little insulin to lower their blood sugar. They eat a peach, their glucose rises, and their pancreas sends out two insulin soldiers to get the insulin out of the blood and into the cells.

You might be insulin-resistant, which means that when you eat a peach, two insulin soldiers can't handle the work, so your body sends out five or six or seven. Your cells effectively close the door when the insulin tries to push glucose into them, so your blood sugar remains high, and your pancreas sends out even more insulin reinforcements. More insulin means more fat storage per peach, Coke, or potato.

You can increase your insulin sensitivity—lessen your fattening response to carbohydrates—by the kind of food you eat and the kind of exercise you do. Gaining lean body mass (muscle) makes you more insulin-sensitive, which helps you get or stay lean by lowering your blood-sugar response to any carbs you eat.

06 Variety is overrated

In the 2.4 million years before the 1400s, everybody ate local foods. If you lived in Africa, you ate local wild game and a few roots, not quinoa or açai berries. If you were an Eskimo, you ate seal liver, polar bears, and fish, not nectarines from Chile in December. Grocery store variety is convenient but unnatural, and it isn't a nutritional requirement.

You might think that your choices will be limited if you give up or severely cut back on carbs, but glance at this list of no-carb and low-carb foods:

NO-CARB AND LOW-CARB FOODS

- Bacon
- Bison
- Ground beef
- Ham
- Liver
- Pulled pork
- Rabbit
- Ribs
- Steak
- Tongue
- Halibut
- Salmon
- Sardines
- Sole
- Clams
- Mussels
- Oysters
- Scallops
- Shrimp
- Chicken
- Rock Cornish game hens
- Turkey
- Eggs
- Blue cheese
- Brie
- Cheddar cheese
- Cottage cheese
- Cowgirl Creamery Mt. Tam cheese
- Gorgonzola cheese
- Mascarpone cheese
- Parmesan cheese
- Provolone cheese
- Whipped cream
- Olive oil
- Tea, coffee

FOODS LOW ENOUGH IN CARBS TO EAT AT ANY MEAL, BUT NOT AT EVERY MEAL EVERY DAY

- Asparagus
- Bell peppers
- Broccoli
- Brussels sprouts
- Coconut
- Collard greens
- Garlic
- Kale
- Macadamia nuts
- Mushrooms
- Olives
- Onions
- Purple cabbage
- Romaine
- Seaweed
- Spinach
- Blueberries, blackberries, raspberries, strawberries
- Tomatoes
- Zucchini
- Dark chocolate (at least 80% cocoa)
- Greek yogurt (plain)

Cook and combine and season them different ways, and you'll have plenty of variety and an ideal diet.

Have a meal of salmon, coconut, collard greens with butter, and macadamias. Serve it to guests—they won't complain about lack of variety. See the list, "Ten dinners, minimal carbs," on page 25.

07 You eat less often when you eat more fat and fewer carbs

This point can't be overstated, but I will try.

We've all heard that it's healthier and better for your weight to eat frequent, smaller meals rather than fewer big ones. The number usually recommended is six small instead of three big. That's nonsense, and is especially bad advice when the recommended small meals and snacks are supposedly healthy foods like fruit, whole grains, carrots, and the odd finger sandwich. Eating small, carb-dense meals will maintain a constant high level of glucose and insulin. It'll prevent you from burning fat and will keep you hungry all day long.

Doubt this? Try it for a week and you'll watch your six small meals a day turn into six medium-sized ones, or possibly three large meals with three snacks in between—and you're thinking "it's fine—six meals a day!" It's not a willpower problem, it's just what happens when you fill yourself with carbohydrates. You get hungry all the time. Instead, cut the carbs and fill up on fat.

08 The dangers of eating too few carbs

There are none. It's unlikely that humans would have evolved to require high doses of carbohydrates, since for 99 percent of our time on Earth—from about 2.5 million years ago to about 11,000 years ago when people learned to plant grains—carbs were scarce, and sometimes virtually absent. Today, there is a minimum requirement for vitamins, minerals, protein, and fat, but not for carbs. Ice agers, Inuits, and others who live in the snowy, icy regions where plants are too scarce to contribute to diet have survived and in fact thrived for hundreds, and in some cases thousands of generations.

In the early 1900s, Norwegian scientist and explorer Vilhjalmur Stefansson lived with the Eskimos for eleven years. For most of the year, his diet was the same as the Inuit—99 percent animal—and he thrived. When he left Alaska and reported his diet to the scientific and medical community, they thought he was lying. They didn't believe that he could be that healthy on an all-meat diet. Stefansson volunteered to live for two years at New York's Bellevue Hospital. His health continued to surpass that of the hospital workers and doctors.

On a carb-scarce diet, your blood sugar will plummet and stabilize at a natural level, and you'll burn your body fat for fuel.

The stresses of modern life and exposure to modern pollutants increase the need for certain nutrients that a pure meat and fat diet might not provide, so be prudent. Take an all-purpose supplement, some omega-3s, eat a few leaves, and you're covered.

09 Too much protein makes you fatter, not stronger

When you eat more protein than your body can use in a few hours, the extra turns into glucose and raises your blood sugar. The rise in blood sugar from eating protein isn't as quick or dramatic as it is when you eat carbs, but it does go up. Think of excess protein as a sort of carbs lite. Get enough, but don't think chomping down pounds of animal muscle will make you stronger. It doesn't work like that.

Thirty grams of protein per meal is about all you can use. That's four and a half eggs, or three eggs plus cheese, a can and a half of sardines, or three to five ounces of beef, twelve slices of bacon. When there's a food label, read it for the protein measure.

If you're a heavily muscled man over 200 pounds and want to grow even more muscles, 100 to 120 grams of protein (5 eggs + 1 cup cottage cheese + 8-ounce steak) a day is enough. If you're not that big and aren't obsessed with size but still want to get stronger, 70 to 80 grams is fine.

Average-sized women do well on 55 to 70 grams of protein a day; petite women, about 45 to 50 grams.

10 Get most of your calories from fat

To burn fat you have to eat fat.

It's not that eating fat in and of itself makes you burn it. It's that carbs and excess protein stop you from burning fat by raising your blood sugar and insulin.

Fat doesn't raise your blood sugar and insulin. But if you combine fat with carbohydrates, the carbs will raise your sugar, the sugar will raise your insulin, the insulin will make you store all those calories (including the fat calories) as body fat. You'll get fat on hamburgers when you eat the buns, too.

Without the carbs, and the glucose and insulin spike that follows, fat becomes a fuel. You burn it up when you move around, and it keeps you from feeling hungry, so you aren't always looking for your next meal.

Odd as it may seem, eating fat not only doesn't make you fat; it is the only way to lose fat.

11 How to eat a sandwich

Throw out the bread, both pieces. You may like the bread or the bun on your sandwich, but think of it as a convenience that keeps your hands clean and your body fat, because that sums it up. The burger or turkey or egg salad filling is the best part anyway—the bread is just a fattening, high-carb handle for it.

The modern world is accommodating. Burger joints won't cry if you don't eat their buns. Reuben sandwiches are nearly as good without the bread—you still get the sauerkraut, pastrami, and cheese, and if you order a Reuben without the bread, the restaurant is likely to give you more pastrami and sauerkraut, because they don't want it to look so small. Win-win.

At home and on your own, use thin-sliced cheese as bread. One slice makes a good hot-dog handle, and two slices make a normal sandwich. If you can't imagine life without sandwiches, make them this way.

12 Get off your lite version of the sumo wrestler weight-gain program

Sumo wrestlers typically weigh more than 400 pounds, about 260 pounds more than the average Japanese man weighs. They get there by eating huge meals of meat, white rice, noodles, and beer, followed by a nap. The glut of carbs and excess protein spike the sumo's blood sugar, and the napping assures that none of the glucose is burned as fuel during exercise.

A typical day's eating in America consists of three light versions of the sumo fattening plan:

- **MORNING:** Bowl of cereal or a muffin with orange juice, followed by a drive to work and sitting at a desk until lunch.
- **LUNCH:** Sandwich, banana, and apple juice, followed by more desk-sitting and maybe a walk down the hall to the meeting room full of chairs. Drive home in the evening.
- **DINNER:** Spaghetti with meatballs, French bread, sparkling apple cider or a beer, followed by a few hours on the sofa or in front of the computer. No exercise to burn off the glucose.

If that's been your strategy, it might be why you weigh too much. Flip it around: Cut the carbs, eat healthy fats, and exercise some—especially after meals—to keep your insulin low. Try this tomorrow:

- **BREAKFAST:** Bacon and eggs or dinner leftovers of meat and greens. Cream or butter in your tea or coffee. Do twenty push-ups or kettlebell swings before getting in the car. It should take you 2 minutes.

- **LUNCH:** Sandwich minus the bread—turkey slices rolled up with cheese, hard-boiled eggs, and some greens or nuts.
- **DINNER:** Meat without potatoes or bread, and a salad without croutons or sweet dressing (only if you feel like eating greens—you don't need them!). Water or one glass of red wine.
- **LATE-NIGHT SNACK OPTION YOU PROBABLY WON'T NEED:** Small bowl of plain Greek yogurt with a handful of macadamias.

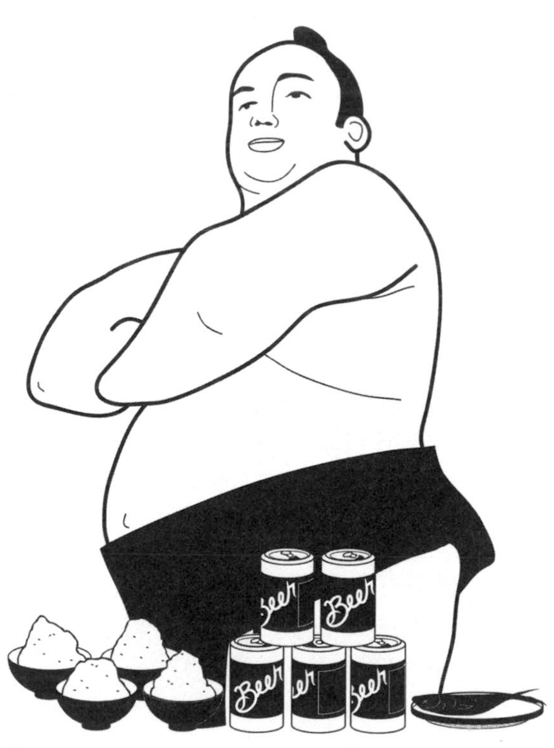

13 Four low-carb diets

THE ATKINS DIET

Robert Atkins wasn't the first high-fat, low-carb champion, but he was the first to reach the masses when he introduced the Atkins Diet in his 1972 book *Dr. Atkins' Diet Revolution*. It has sold millions of copies and has many spin-offs, but along the way has become—unfairly but understandably—the poster diet for those who fear being fat. In retrospect, Atkins should have emphasized low carb as much as high fat.

The first two weeks of the Atkins Diet, called the induction phase, is ketogenic, defined below, by design—you're limited to 20 grams of carbs or less per day, which induces ketosis and suppresses hunger. Over the next several weeks and months, you get to up your carbs a little, but the foundation is still high fat, super low carb.

The most recent Atkins book, *The New Atkins For a New You*, was published in 2010, seven years after Atkins died (by Drs. Westman, Phinney, and Volek, all of whom have written their own low-carb diet manuals). It's a rational, more scientific, less in-your-face version of the original; it de-emphasizes the amounts of cream and quantities of food Atkins promised you could eat, and it arms you against high-fat/low-carb detractors better than the original did.

Those detractors like to point out that Atkins died from his own diet, but that's not true. When he was seventy-two (in 2003), he slipped on some ice and hit his head, causing internal bleeding. He almost died in the ambulance, and was in the ICU for a couple of weeks.

He retained a lot of fluid, gained almost 60 pounds, and eventually died of organ failure unrelated to his diet.

THE PALEO DIET

This diet went public in 2002, with the publication of Loren Cordain's book *The Paleo Diet*. Loren Cordain is a professor of health and science, and has a special interest in Stone Age diets.

Cordain's Paleo Diet allows lean meats, unlimited fresh fruits and nonstarchy vegetables, lots of nuts, and now and then a diet soda. No dairy, no grains, no fatty meats. Compared to the other diets here, it allows more carbs and less fat, and is the easiest to follow if you're coming off a standard diet that includes bread and pasta. The Paleo Diet is less strict than the others; it's a good starter diet and it may be all you need.

THE PRIMAL BLUEPRINT DIET

This, like most of the low-carb diets, is high in fat, more like Atkins than Paleo. The Primal Blueprint Diet was introduced and named by Mark Sisson, a former triathlete, author, and one of the best voices to come out of the anticarb movement. Mark's blog is the curiously named Mark's Daily Apple, and he's done as much for the low-carb/high-fat movement as anybody, and maybe more. He is the one who turned me around, and remains a hero to me.

The Primal Blueprint Diet eliminates grains, but allows and encourages fatty meats, saturated fats, and a little fatty dairy. It's about 80 percent fat. If you like everything about the Atkins diet but all that cream grosses you out, try the Primal Blueprint Diet.

A KETOGENIC DIET

Ketones are naturally occurring molecules that provide energy if and when your insulin levels drop to the point where glucose is not being provided to the cells. When your blood sugar drops and your insulin level follows, you are no longer able to supply glucose to your cells. You start to burn fat and produce ketones for energy. The three ketone bodies present in your blood when you're in ketosis are acetone (like the solvent), acetoacetate, and beta-hydroxybutyrate.

A ketogenic diet is a super low-carb diet that lowers your glucose level to the point at which your body effectively gives up on glucose and starts to burn fat and produce ketones as an alternative—and that means you are "in ketosis." Burning ketones makes your body work for you as the efficient machine it was meant to be.

The Atkins, Paleo, or Primal Blueprint diets may be incidentally ketogenic, but *intentionally* ketogenic diets—whose main goal is to switch your fuel source to ketones—tend to have even more fat, less protein, and fewer carbs.

Beware of the claim that "Any diet will work if you stick to it." That lie is based on the myth that losing weight is a matter of eating fewer calories than you burn up, and ignores the effects of insulin on fat storage and hunger. It would be convenient if there were dozens of diets that worked, so that you could find the one that allowed your favorite foods and snacks, and still win the fat war, but it doesn't work that way. Diets that don't limit carbs, yet require smaller portions and more exercise, are doomed to fail because they keep you hungry and make you store fat.

Effective diets will minimize your insulin, which will reduce your fat storage and make you get calories from your existing body fat, which will minimize hunger. Diets that do that may not be billed as ketogenic diets, but to some degree they probably are.

14 You need food, not a pyramid or a plate

The government has been advising us on what to eat and how much for more than a hundred years, dumbing it down for us in a series of wheels, charts, and pyramids. The early charts and wheels allowed healthy amounts of meat, butter, and fats. But by anti-carb standards, there was still far too much bread, cereal, and potatoes. Fear of fat and beef took hold in the 1970s, and the famous Food Pyramid embodied that by putting bread, cereal, rice, or pasta as the basis of every meal. Adult obesity rates skyrocketed in 1990—just about the time the kids who were born in the 1970s had time to become adults and gain weight from eating the way the government told them to.

In 2011, the Food Pyramid was officially replaced by MyPlate, which has no mention of fats. Presumably there are some in the protein and the side dish of dairy, but since we're told to avoid saturated fats (all dairy fats are saturated) you're probably meant to interpret the dairy to mean nonfat milk, yogurt, and cottage cheese. Since fat is so important to your health—as it is the only nutrient that doesn't raise insulin—its absence is evidence that something's wrong with MyPlate.

Food is a political issue, and politicians hoping for a long career in politics aren't going to endorse an agenda that makes it hard to sell wheat, corn, or potatoes.

Here are some guidelines that work better than MyPlate:

NEVER: Grains, soda, fruit juice, sweets.

NOW AND THEN: Roots that aren't fluffy potatoes. Whole fruit. Nuts and seeds.

WHENEVER YOU FEEL LIKE 'EM: Above-ground vegetables, especially leaves and especially dark leaves. It's not that they're so full of accessible nutrients; it's that they're high in water and low in carbs, and that the carbs they have are bound up in cellulose, so they aren't fully digestible. Indigestible carbs can feed your gut bacteria (a good thing, see page 154).

LOTS: Young, fatty, oily fish—herring, wild salmon, sardines, and trout from the coldest waters. Eggs. Mammal meat, especially fatty meats from grass-fed or wild animals. Cheese, cream, butter, macadamia nuts, olive and coconut oils.

15 The most important meal of the day . . . to skip

Ask the next dozen strangers you see, "What's the most important meal of the day?" If they've been properly brainwashed by the grain-sellers, they'll say breakfast. When you're a carb-eater, your body's nocturnal activity involves burning sugar for 7 to 8 hours, so by morning your stomach will be growling for you to put something into it. If you skip breakfast, your blood sugar might be too low by late morning, and you'll feel starved, maybe lethargic, and definitely desperate for food. That's why, for a sugar-burner, breakfast *is* the most important meal of the day.

It's different for a fat-burner. Since you're adapted to getting your energy from fat, your blood sugar doesn't spike and fall off the cliff the way a sugar-burner's does. It's far more stable, and you don't wake up rarin' to dive into a high-carb breakfast.

The pull of ritualistic eating is still there, but it's different from the desperation hunger of a sugar-burner. You can satisfy the ritual with fatty coffee or tea, which keeps your blood sugar low enough to keep you burning fat until lunch or even beyond. Then eat a fatty burger with cheese and bacon for lunch, and you'll cruise into the evening, no hunger, no problem.

16 Ten dinners, minimal carbs

These are stealth low-carb dinners that you don't have to introduce as "low-carb" because they look normal enough. Every ingredient contributes something—fat, protein, color, crunch, and flavor—but with carb levels low enough to keep you burning fat.

1 Baked or fried salmon, with sautéed chard, and cheese and macadamia nuts for dessert.

2 Bacon burgers with cheese and a salad.

3 Lamb stew meat sautéed in butter or ghee, topped with blue cheese, and a side of plain Greek yogurt with macadamia nuts.

4 Almond-flour coated chicken fried in butter or ghee, with sautéed-in-butter chard, and shredded Parmesan cheese.

5 Super Cobb salad with blue cheese or olive oil and vinegar dressing fortified with broccoli and extra bacon or other meat.

6 Scallops wrapped in bacon and fried in bacon grease, with sautéed broccolini, and soft-boiled eggs on the side.

7 Liver, onions, and bacon sautéed in bacon grease, with plain, full-fat Greek yogurt mixed with crumbled blue cheese on the side, macadamia nuts for dessert.

8 Village-style Greek salad of cucumbers, bell peppers, onions, feta cheese, olives, tomatoes, with sautéed chicken with the skin.

9 Omelet stuffed with Parmesan, red onions, sautéed mushrooms, with a few sheets of dried nori (seaweed).

10 Fatty wieners or bratwurst split lengthwise and fried in butter till they're curly and their skins are crisp and blackish in the places that touch the pan most, with steamed sauerkraut and strong, grainy brown mustard. Yum.

FOOD PARTICULARS

Now that you know that sugar is bad because it spikes your insulin, and fat is good because it doesn't spike your insulin *and* it fills you up, the food recommendations you're about to read will make sense. Some of them will bum you out or make you defensive, and if your family fortune was made on grandpa's fruit orchards or you own a whole grain bakery, you'll probably hate the messenger. My intention is only to steer you away from the foods that make you sick and fat, and toward the ones that fill you up and allow you to burn your own body fat, so you get lean.

By the end of this chapter, you'll have a good feel for what those foods are, and there will be surprises along the way.

Now a word about beer and wine. Red wine has fewer carbs than white wine, and light beer has fewer than regular beer. At the end of the day (literally, when you're ready to go to bed), it's the total carbs you've injested that counts, not their source. Bread or red wine; but best not both.

17 The good fats

Not carbs and not even protein—only fats—have zero effect on blood sugar and insulin. But some fats are healthy and some are deadly. One measure of a healthy fat is its ratio of omega-6 to omega-3 fatty acids. Both are essential for life, but they must be supplied by your diet because your body doesn't make them, and the ratio of omega-6 to omega-3 fatty acids is key. When omega-6 fatty acids dominate in a ratio of 20 to 1 or more, which is typical in a normal high-carb diet, your risk rises for obesity, diabetes, high blood pressure, heart disease, asthma, and lots of other diseases of inflammation.

The good fats are:

- cold-water fish fat from salmon, sardines, herring, anchovies; shellfish like crab, shrimp, scallops, and oysters that eat low on the food chain and die young so they don't have time to accumulate mercury the way big old predator fish like tuna and swordfish do. These are high in omega-3s, low in omega-6s.
- animal fat from grass-fed animals. They also have a good ratio of omega-3s to omega-6s, although not as overwhelmingly good as oily fish.
- monounsaturated fats from olives, avocados, and especially macadamia nuts. These aren't high in omega-3s, but they have better omega-6 to omega-3 ratios than do most fatty foods. For instance: olive oil (10 to 1), avocados (15 to 1), macadamia nuts (1 to 1). The numbers for olive oil and avocados look unimpressive until you consider that the ratios for safflower, sesame, and almond oils are 1,000 to 1 or higher. The dominant type of fat in

both olive oil and avocado oil is monounsaturated, which provides health benefits that make up for the unimpressive ratios for omega-3s to omega 6s.

- medium-chain triglycerides (MCTs). These fats are good because they are metabolized differently than other fats. They're easier to burn as energy, and when you do that you make ketones, an efficient fuel for body, heart, and brain functions. By far the best source of MCTs is coconut oil.

WHERE FISH HIGH IN OMEGA-3 FATTY ACIDS GET THEIR OMEGA-3S

Small fish like sardines and herring eat the omega-3 rich algae, bigger fish eat the small fish, you eat the bigger fish. The omega-3s accumulate with each step up the chain, with oily fish like sardines, herring, mackerel, salmon, and tuna ending up being rich with them. It used to be that wild salmon had a great advantage over farmed salmon because farmed salmon didn't have a source of food that provided omega-3 fatty acids. But now the fish farmers feed their salmon formulas high in omega-3s, and in some cases farmed salmon are running neck and neck with wild salmon. Sardines, herring, and mackerel are even better sources of omega-3s than salmon, but most people prefer salmon.

18 The bad fats

It's easy to avoid these entirely; you just have to pay attention.

- Trans fats: In 1902, German scientist Wilhelm Normann—the father of trans fats—knew that saturated fat holds more hydrogen than liquid unsaturated fat, so he figured out a way to add hydrogen to cottonseed oil to make it saturated (solid at room temperature). Any vegetable oil can be hydrogenated, but in the United States, we use mostly soybean oil.

Who benefits from trans fats? Mostly high-volume, cost-conscious cooks and bakers, because trans fats are inexpensive, impart no flavor, and have a shelf life of a year or more even out of the refrigerator. They make extra crispy fried chicken, French fries, and croissants. Trans fats allow salad dressings and margarine to sit around in the jar for months without going rancid.

But once they're in your body, trans fats raise the bad kind of LDL that clogs arteries, and lowers the good kind of cholesterol—HDL—that cleans arteries out. Margarine is a trans-fat product that is far worse for you than the butter it was invented to replace. When moms in the '60s kept a tub of Crisco around as a "healthy" alternative to butter in their homemade cakes and cookies, they were simply swayed by the advertising. It's too late to blame them now, or to lay any guilt on Normann's progeny.

- Seed oils: Sunflower seeds, safflower seeds, sesame seeds, cottonseeds, and rapeseeds are all too high in omega-6 fatty acids. You might think flaxseed oil is good because it is high in omega-3s, but unfortunately, it's not in a form that's as usable to your body as the omega-3s that come from animals, although it doesn't do the harm that the popular seed oils do.

- Soybean oil, corn oil, peanut oil, almond oil, and any other vegetable oil not listed under the "good fats." They're high in omega-6 fats, which are easily damaged by heat and exposure to air, and when damaged, they become even more of an artery clogging threat.

When I say avoid almond oil, I am not saying avoid almonds. When the oil is in the nut, it is part of a whole package that includes other nutrients, and the oil in the nut is protected against oxidation, which brings out the worst in omega-6 oils.

Even on a healthy near-zero–carb diet, you'll get plenty of omega-6 fats, because they're hard to avoid. But the idea is to improve the ratio of omega-3 fats to omega-6 fats in your diet. The best way to do this is to stick with oily fish, grass-fed meat and dairy, and olive, avocado, macadamia, and coconut oils. But just to be sure, take omega-3 supplements—a 1,200 milligram capsule costs less than another 8 ounces of crab or even 3 ounces of cheap canned herring, a personal favorite.

19 Keep your fats cool, or at least don't let them smoke

Fats are healthiest and taste best when they haven't reached the smoke point—which means the point where you see a little bit of smoke. Overheating and reheating fats can form toxins as well as kill off the antioxidants in the oil. For simplicity's sake, the first thing to do is eliminate all the bad fats that I listed previously and focus on these, listed with their approximate smoke points.

Bacon grease	250°F
Butter	300°–370°F
Coconut oil (unrefined)	350°F
Extra virgin olive oil	375°F
Macadamia oil	410°F
Beef fat	420°F
Lard (made from boiling pig fat)	420°F
Ghee	470°F

If adding beef fat and lard to your food or frying pan feels wrong to you, just rule them out and go on to other good ones. And macadamia oil costs too much, so out it goes, too. Here's a sensible approach:

BACON GREASE: Fry eggs in it if it's already in the pan from having just fried bacon; otherwise use ghee or butter.

GHEE, BUTTER, COCONUT OIL: Use for all other meats and for sautéing vegetables; and for fattening up your hot morning beverage.

OLIVE OIL: If a Mediterranean recipe demands it, use olive oil. For salads, too. If you love the taste, splash it unheated onto any cooked food.

There you go. Time and exposure to light can degrade fats and make them less healthy, so besides keeping them cool, store them in dark jars or cupboards, and eat them soon—within about a month.

20 Drink a fatty breakfast

Put three or four tablespoons of butter, ghee, cream, and/or coconut oil in your morning tea or coffee. This is a perfect breakfast.

If you're just starting out on the low-carb way of life and still crave solid food in the morning, replace that muffin and coffee with two or three eggs and four or five slices of bacon along with your tea or coffee. As you get into ketosis, you'll find you're not so hungry when you wake up and won't need all that food until later in the day.

Once you get over not eating in the morning, a hot fatty drink like this will feel normal, even indulgent. And it really works. Pouring hot, healthy, melted fat into your stomach isn't as immediately satisfying as forking into a stack of flapjacks oozing with maple syrup, but it's not the ascetic opposite, either. The goal here isn't to fool yourself into feeling satisfied when you aren't—that's the sugar-burner's game. The trick is to become a fat-burner who is satisfied with a high-fat, zero-carb breakfast and to avoid cravings for sugar, sugar, sugar.

21 The whole grains ruse

No food has as diversified a fan club as whole grains. They're eaten by jocks, Eastern mystics and religious leaders, hippies, the poor, the rich, and are fully endorsed by the U.S. Food and Drug Administration, the American Diabetes Association, the American Heart Association, and most doctors, nurses, nutritionists, and others who don't understand the insidious harm they can do.

I know there are populations of people around the world who subsist mainly on whole grains and manage to stay skinny, but they're hardworking farmers or mountain people who work long days outside, and burn up glucose faster than the average semisedentary American does. And they don't eat as much. In Japan, a serving of white rice is the size of half a tennis ball, and they don't go back for seconds and thirds. They also don't eat between meals. Many Americans eat pretty much all day long, with spikes in the morning, at noon, and in the evening. Whole grains for them are a different game in another league.

To some people, the word *fiber* suggests a scrubbing, cleansing, scouring of fat from your arteries and colon, but fiber doesn't scrub anything. Your digestive system can't extract much nutrition from it, so its main "contribution" is larger and more frequent bowel movements, which wouldn't be necessary if the fibrous bran weren't so indigestible. And the digestible part (technically, the endosperm that makes up 85 percent of the grain's volume) turns into sugar, jacks up your insulin, and makes you fatter and less healthy.

General Mills has been calling Cheerios (even the dulce de leche and chocolate varieties) "heart healthy"—because of the fiber—for more than a decade. Hard-core whole-grainers would argue that sugar-infused whole grains shouldn't be lumped together with unadulterated ones. I'd take it another step and point out that to your blood, even natural, unsugared whole grains jack up your sugar and keep you hungry for more of it. Their reputation as healthy makes them the "friend" who's out to get you.

WHOLE GRAINS ARE STILL GRAINS, AND HUMANS DON'T HAVE THE DIGESTIVE SYSTEM FOR THEM.

Following is a list of whole grains, with their carbohydrate content in dry weight. Since there are about 454 grams in a pound, and white rice is 73 percent carbs, this translates to 454 grams × 0.81 = 331 grams of carbs in a 1-pound bag—a whole week's worth of carbs if you're being careful to eat few carbs. Once you've started eating grains—a mound of rice, a piece of bread, a bowl of granola—it's pretty hard to stop. They keep you coming back, arguably more than most other foods.

Grain	% Carbohydrate (grams in dry weight)
Amaranth	66
Barley	73
Brown rice	76
Buckwheat	70
Corn	74
Millet	73
Oats	66

Quinoa 69
Rye 69
Triticale 67
Whole wheat 73
Wild rice 75

Of course, you don't eat grains dry. You cook them and they soak up water, which makes them more digestible and less filling, so you eat more at a sitting. Water or not, it's still a carb-heavy meal that raises your glucose and insulin and makes you store more fat.

Non–meat eaters consider some whole grains a good source of protein, but they're good sources only if you compare them to fruits and vegetables. Throw animal products into the equation for comparison and grains squirm away in shame. Even when you combine them to supply all the essential amino acids for complete protein, the carb load in grains will make you fat and keep you hungry way before the protein in them does you any good.

Combining two or three sources of incomplete proteins to make a complete protein seems a strange way to solve the problem. It's better to let the animals with digestive systems for grains eat the grains and convert them into high-quality protein for you to eat.

22 All corn is candy corn

Although most people think of corn as a vegetable—because you can grow it in your garden and it's not sweet like an apricot—it is certainly not a vegetable. It's an especially sugary grain that's been monkeyed with more than most foods. It began as something called teosinte, a cornlike grain that grew in what's now Mexico. It wasn't consumed in the quantities corn is today. It was tiny, lacked a cob, and the few kernels it produced were hard, like the Indian corncobs you see around Thanksgiving. You didn't just rip off a stalk of teosinte and start gnawing.

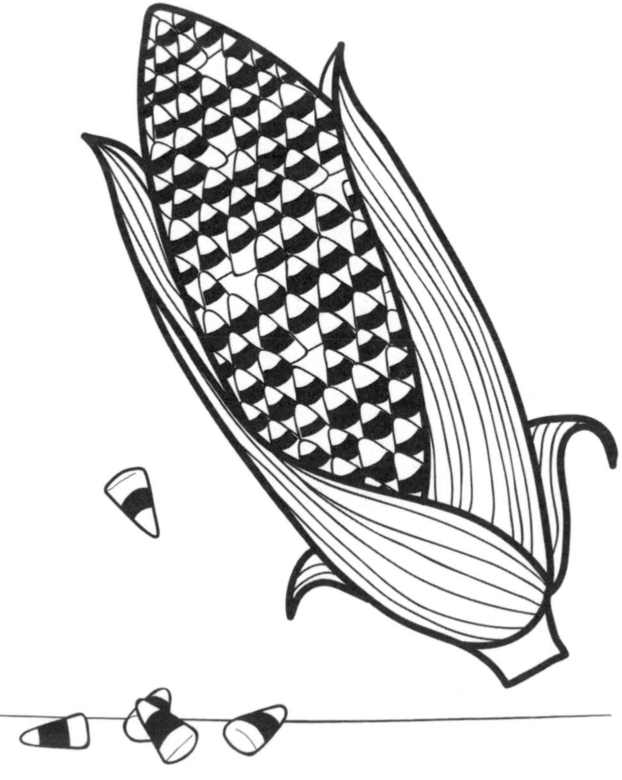

Then, about 6,400 years ago, farmers selectively bred the thickest, fullest plants, and over the next many centuries it became maize, a single-cob plant that any modern kid would call corn. He wouldn't eat it though—not soft or sweet enough. But in the early 1960s, midwestern Americans took over.

Today's supersweet hybrid corn was developed in the labs at the University of Illinois in the '60s, and is the parent of high-fructose corn syrup, the main sweetener in the most fattening foods still legal to sell. Beef ranchers feed cattle a less sweet variety of corn to fatten them for market, but we people get the sweetest corn of all, and the high glucose spikes and fat storage that come with it.

Corn chips, corn on the cob, creamed corn, corn bread, corn pone, corn chowder, steamed corn, corn flakes—avoid them all. Halloween candy corn—almost entirely corn syrup—is at least obviously candy, so you know you're supposed to avoid it. Everyday corn, because it's promoted as a healthy whole food, is more dangerous because you gobble it up in mouthfuls of sweet kernels or mush. At your next picnic, if you're given a cob of corn, slather it with butter and slurp it off. Do that a few times, and then drop the yellow menace in the dirt, so you don't have to be sneaky when you toss it in the trash, where it can't hurt you. It goes to waist or it goes to waste, depending on where you put it.

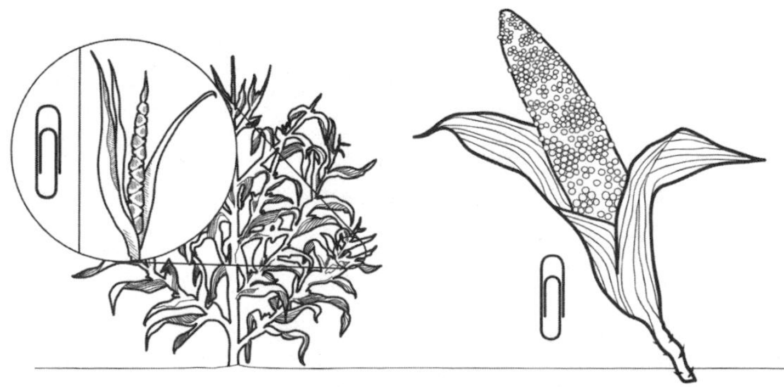

23 The fruit ruse

Before agriculture, fruit was seasonal, small, sweet only when compared to meat and greens, and rare. Now it's selectively bred to be huge, supersweet, and abundant; and no matter where you live, you can buy South American grapes in November. Fruits are universally considered natural and healthy, but compared to their ancient relatives, today's fruits are pretty much just juicy sugar orbs that, from a health perspective, look good only when compared to grains and donuts. With a few exceptions, fruit is the ultimate trick food, a "devil in disguise." Read this out loud: "Fruit makes me fat."

It's not just the quantity of sugar, but the kind. Glucose, lactose, sucrose, and other sugars get metabolized (used as fuel) all over your body, but fruit sugar—fructose—goes straight to your liver. Since your liver didn't evolve to handle huge doses of fructose, it turns it into triglycerides (dangerous fat) and sends it out into your blood, to your arteries, and onto your hips. High-fructose corn syrup is particularly fattening because it's 55 percent fructose (converts to lots of triglycerides), and 41 percent glucose (jacks up insulin).

If you have a weight problem now, it's more likely due to grains than to whole fruit. Between the two, eat the fruit, since it is mostly water and therefore less concentrated. But adding fruit in any of its forms—dried, fresh, or juiced—to a diet that already includes grains is pouring gas on a fire. After you give up grains, give up dried fruit, then fruit juice, then fresh fruit. It's fine to stick with berries and avocados, because they're the lowest in carbohydrates of all the sweet fruits.

24 In vegetables, darker is bitterer is better

Dark, leafy vegetables tend to have more nutrients and taste more bitter than lighter vegetables that grow in heads, like cabbages and iceberg lettuce, and here's why: Exposure to the sun stresses the plant, and triggers a defense response in the form of plant compounds that we consider to be nutrients—vitamins, minerals, and antioxidants—but whose primary purpose is to protect the plant from insects and the sun. They're not there just to invigorate you. The next time you go to the produce section of the grocery store or to your farmers' market, look for broad, flat, pale green leaves; you won't find 'em, and it's for the same reason that you don't find fair complexions native to Africa. Dark leaves, like dark skin, evolved to fend off the sun. The palest leaves are on the inner layers of head lettuces, protected from the sun deep in a physical barrier, with no need to be bitter because pests and the sun can't get to them, anyway. And there's no need for these leaves to develop sunscreens, because they live in the dark, like those blind albino newts that live in the caves in Borneo about 2,000 feet underground. The inner leaves of any lettuce or cabbage (including Brussels sprouts) are the lightest and mildest.

Broad, exposed leaves like kale, endive, collards, chard, spinach, watercress, dandelion greens, and mustard greens reach for the sun and lay out flat like a 1950s sunbather. That exposure helps them develop phytonutrients and antioxidants that protect them from pests. The phytonutrients give them their familiar, bitter taste that most kids hate but adults have learned to tolerate—no doubt in part because they feel virtuous eating them.

Whether the leaves are shrouded and light and mild, or flat and dark and bitter, they're a good part of life and add color, variety, and texture to any meal. It's unlikely that you can extract all of their nutrients from their largely indigestible cellulose, but those nutrients evolved to protect the plant, anyway, not to infuse you with health. Over time and with effort, you can learn to like the strong taste of some of the healthier greens, and that is not a bad thing.

25 Never order an egg white omelet

The yolk is the best part of the egg. It's 50 percent of the egg's protein and all of its fat. Most people think the cholesterol in the yolk will clog your arteries, but it won't. The fat in the yolk is healthy as long as you don't mix it with carbs, and it's the most filling part of the omelet. You can eat egg white omelets all day long and never feel satisfied. I've done it. Whole-egg omelets are filling because they're fatty. Yolk-only omelets would be better still, but let's be reasonable.

Yolks get a bad rap because they contain cholesterol, but there is no relationship between cholesterol in the egg yolk and the cholesterol clogging your arteries. High bad-cholesterol numbers are driven by carbohydrates and omega-6 oils, not the healthy fats in egg yolks.

26 Crack your own nuts

The normal rap on nuts is they're too fatty, but when you *want* most of your calories to come from fat, that's not a problem. Almonds, peanuts, walnuts, and filberts make the low-carb team, but they're not starters. The problem is that they're cheap and easy to overeat, and they're too high in omega-6 oils for a weight loss diet. Curb your nut eating by buying them in the shell whenever possible. That will help limit you to about ten almonds, maybe eight walnuts, and at most twenty-five peanuts. Shelled, you might eat triple those figures.

If you love nuts, empty your piggy bank and spring for macadamias. They have fewer omega-6 fats than any other nut, and since we have too much omega-6 fats in our diets, the tiny omega-6 load in macadamias is a good thing. They're also the highest in fat and lowest in carbs, and even though they're sold shelled, they are expensive enough that you won't power down handfuls of them as though they were beer nuts at a bar. Keep them in the freezer so they'll be cold and crunchy. On a super low-carb diet, it doesn't take many macadamias to fill you up. The trick is to put the bag back in the freezer after a few fingertipsful, and give your gut time to register them—20 minutes will do it. If you eat nuts or any other fatty food, stop before you're full. If you keep eating until you're full, you'll be overeating for about 20 minutes.

The one nut you'll most want to avoid is the terrifying Brazil nut. I love them, but they have a high concentration of selenium, an overdose of which has unpleasant side effects, including brittle hair that falls out, loose fingernails, dizziness, difficult breathing, stomach pains, and irritability. Two-thirds of a Brazil nut has all the selenium you need for a day. More balanced sources of selenium are—no surprise—fish, meat, poultry, and eggs.

Here's a confession: In the old days when I feared fat and had swallowed the fiber Kool-Aid, I'd eat peanuts—shell and all—hoping to surround the fat I consumed with fiber and make it less accessible. At my worst, I'd eat only the shells.

27 Olive oil is good, but not God

Olive oil is high in monounsaturated fats—those are good for you—and being a fat, doesn't spike your glucose and insulin. Most olive oil fans advise you to get only the "extra virgin" kind, which means the oil is cold-pressed from the olive without using heat or solvents, and the oil that oozes out has a lower acidity than other types of olive oil. It tastes mild off the spoon, but you might not be able to tell if it were tossed in a complicated salad with lots of other flavors and textures.

Store olive oil in a dark place, and below about 72°F. It'll keep longer that way, but the idea is to eat it up, anyway. Mix it with plain or balsamic vinegar (The vinegar has a few carbs, but if you've recently cut out all grains and fruit, allow yourself this temporary vestige of your pre–low-carb life. Eventually you can use plain vinegar, which has zero carbs and tastes good enough.) and add tomatoes. Freeze the mixture in an ice cube tray and suck on the cubes when you want to eat but are not hungry—it makes an interesting treat, especially when a friend asks you what you're sucking on. Consume it however you want, but preferably unheated. You want to cook with it? OK, fine, as long as you don't let it smoke. Just don't cook with it as a healthier alternative to pastured butter, ghee, or coconut oil, because it's not. It's just another good fat.

28 God is a coconut

Coconut is right up there with salmon in the "not magic, but damn close to it" category, partly because it's so low in carbs for a nonleafy plant, but mainly because it's such a great source of medium-chain triglycerides (MCTs). Coconut oil is 66 percent MCTs. MCTs are fat royalty because they aren't stored in the body the way other fats are. They're readily burned as energy and, in the burning, produce more ketones (cell fuel alternative to glucose) than any other kind of fat. MCTs are being used in treatments for obesity, cancer, Alzheimer's, Parkinson's, and other neurological diseases that typically rely on a steady supply of glucose.

MCTs aren't easy to come by, and coconut products, especially coconut oil, have far more of it than any other food.

Pure coconut oil, the cheapest source of those great MCTs, costs about $10 a pint, cheap enough to eat or drink every day, and is available plain and flavored. Put it in hot drinks or eat it right off the spoon if you're up to it. Better yet, make your own chocolate with it (see recipe for Breakfast Chocolate, page 206).

Coconut butter—sometimes called "coconut cream"—is whipped-up coconut solids. You can make it yourself, or buy it from the pros for about the same price as coconut oil. It's not as high in MCTs as the oil because it's not *pure* fat, but it's not as weird to eat straight, and once you get used to it, it's delicious.

Coconut milk is juiced coconut meat. It's white like normal milk, so you expect more flavor, but alas, it tastes like thick white water. On the plus side, it has only 1 to

2 grams of carbs per 8 ounces. If you demand more flavor, sweeten it with a sweetener like stevia or Truvia.

Coconut water is the liquid inside a raw coconut, and is all the rage these days, because it's so sweet. It costs about $2 a pint, and has too many carbs for me, but if you're weaning yourself off fruit juice and Coke, it's a good transitional drink. If you love it but don't want to guzzle it, drink it only straight from the coconut. Get a whole coconut, shake it to verify that there's still water inside. Drill or ream out two of the three holes (to prevent dribbling), then tilt and suck out the sweet water.

Dried coconut—shredded or flaked, raw or toasted—is the foundation of good cereal (see page 198) and trail-mixy stuff, and is good for texture and taste in low-carb desserts. Of course, buy only unsweetened. If you're cleaning out your cabinet and can't part with your bag of sweetened flaked coconut, wash it in a colander a couple of times and you'll remove most of the sugar.

Shredded or flaky coconut is great for fake cereal and in homemade chocolate (see page 206), and if, despite my attempt to wrestle you away from fiber obsession, you still like the idea of a little fiber to keep things passing through, coconut "meat" in any form is a good way to get it without the carb load of grains.

29 How to get a figure like a potato

Just eat them. And if you're going to eat potatoes, what the hell, go the extra inch and eat French fries, because there's just not that much difference. On a bad-for-you scale, one's a 98, the other's a 109. On a "good-for-you" scale, one's a minus 20, the other minus 25. So really, take your pick.

People have been eating roots for millions of years, but always as a poor substitute for meat or a vehicle for tasty seasonings of questionable benefit. Even when potatoes are allowed to remain unprocessed, they're a far cry from the ancient roots eaten by early humans and still today by people who live in hidden jungles and on mountaintops. Those wild roots are small, misshapen, tough, are high in indigestible fiber with almost no sugar to sweeten them up, and have to be found underground and dug up with a stick. Traipsing around the tangled slopes for the better part of a day looking for them to dig up, and then sharing your meager bounty with the rest of the clan at suppertime, won't make you fat.

Modern roots are sometimes still shaped like haywire, but more often they're big and oblong, tender and sweet, and you can put pounds of them into your shopping cart with a couple of sweeps of your arm. Russet potatoes are the worst. You can bake and glaze them or mash them and serve roots that taste like candy and don't even require chewing. Maybe you've heard of the Glycemic Index (GI), a measurement of how much a food raises your glucose (and therefore, insulin) levels. The higher a food's GI score, the more it jacks up blood sugar, and according to the index, a 5-ounce russet spikes your glucose as much as a pint of Coke. Yams and sweet potatoes aren't as bad, but no roots can do as much good for you as leaves or meat, so go easy on all roots and stay away from russets entirely.

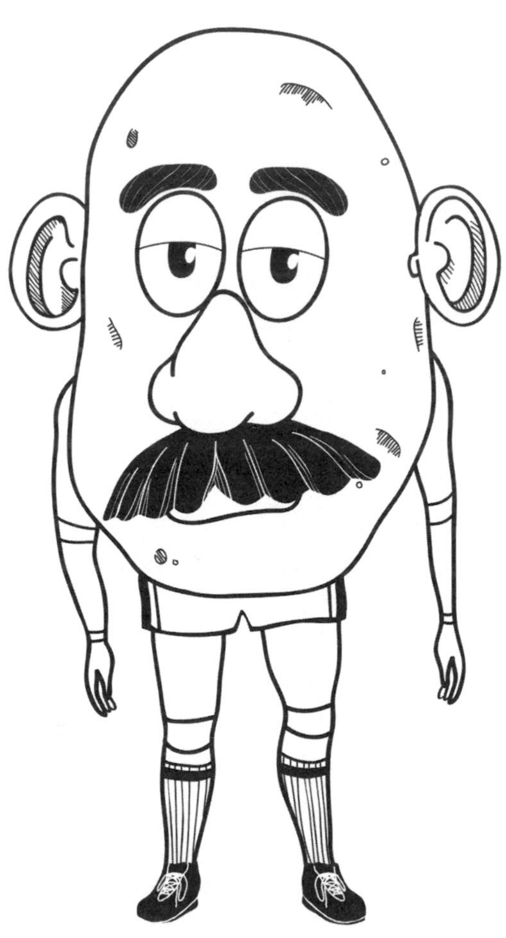

30 Salt and blood pressure, simplified

When you eat too many pickles, pretzels, chips, or sauerkraut your fingers swell because they're salty and salt makes you retain water. Nobody dies from swollen fingers, but the extra volume enters your arteries, like putting more water in a water balloon. The water balloon responds by getting bigger, which keeps the pressure inside stable, although the walls of the balloon get thinner, and may burst. Your arteries have an antibursting response: They grow thicker muscles on the inside, which crams the blood into a smaller area, raising your blood pressure.

If your arteries are clean, the increased restriction is no big deal. But typically, people who eat tons of salt also eat tons of carbs and bad fats that coat the artery walls with plaque—a fat-based substance. And that's a problem. The high-pressure gushing blood can rip off a chunk or flap, exposing gooey fat underneath it, forming a clot that can lead to a ruptured artery, stroke, or heart attack. Without the fat there, your arteries are wide open, so your blood flows like cool, clear water through a fat plastic straw.

Happily, on a super low-carb diet—a ketogenic diet (see pages 20–21)—you excrete more sodium, potassium, and magnesium in your urine, and should replace it by diet, including pickles and sauerkraut, but no pretzels or chips.

LOW BLOOD PRESSURE

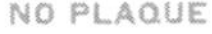

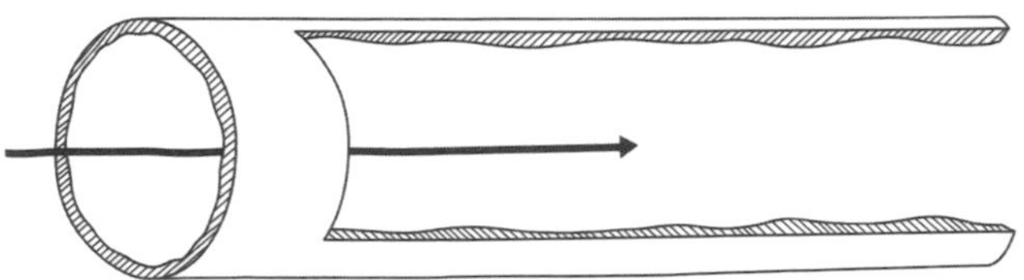

HIGH BLOOD PRESSURE
NO PLAQUE

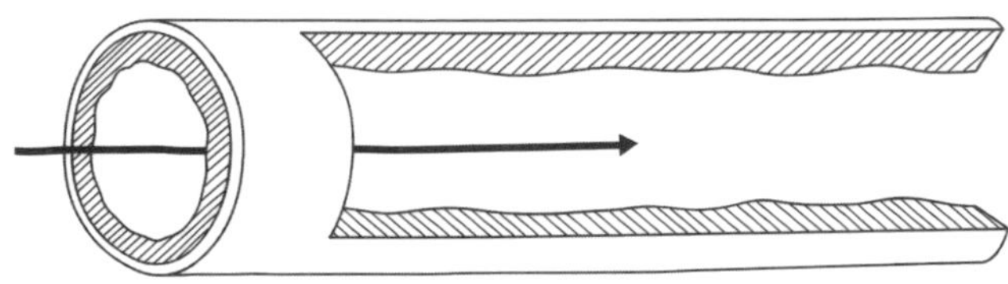

HIGH BLOOD PRESSURE
PLUS PLAQUE

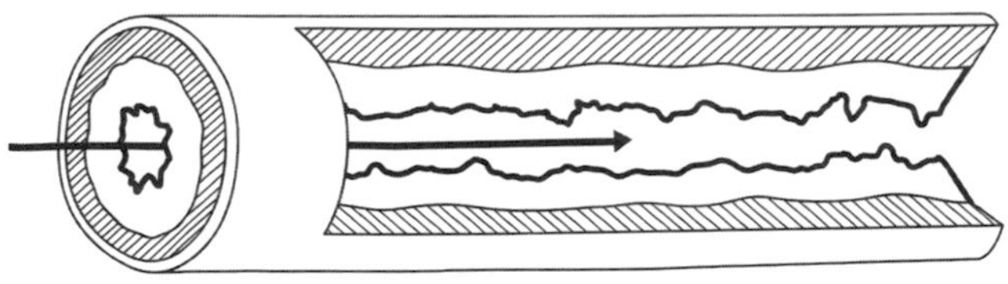

BIRTH OF A BLOOD CLOT

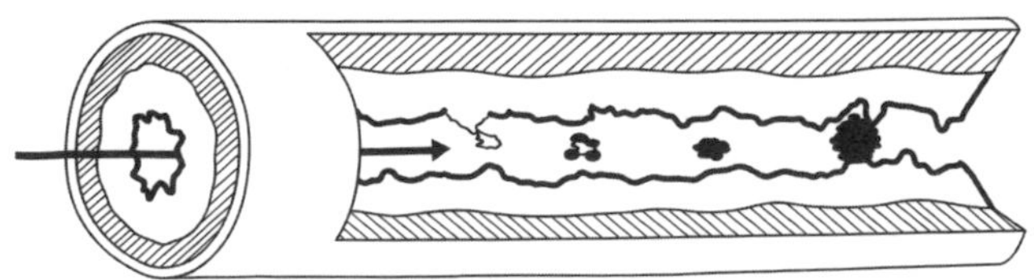

31 Soybeans: The honeymoon is over; the nutrition is overrated

Soybeans were the hippies' salvation in the 1970s and '80s when everybody but ranchers and Atkins disciples thought meat was immoral and red meat was deadly. But now that we know better (and we do), there's no health-based reason to eat soy in any form, and some really good reasons not to.

Soy is an "antinutrient" due to its high concentrations of phytic acid, which reduces your body's ability to use iron, zinc, copper, and magnesium, and increases your requirement of vitamins D and B-12 (neither of which soy provides).

Menopausal women are often advised to up their intake of soy, because it contains phytoestrogens, which mimic the effects of the natural estrogen they lose as they age. Whether this minor effect is fair compensation for its antinutrient properties is up to the patient and doctor to figure out, but if you're an adult man or an infant, it's best to stay away from food and supplements high in female hormones.

Soy's trump card has always been its protein, which is about 50 percent of its dry weight. It trounces all other plant sources of protein, but that's like being the best ballet dancer in the coal mine. If it's protein you're after, meat is your friend.

32 Greek yogurt or none at all

Greek yogurt is regular yogurt that's been drained of some of its juicy whey to make it thicker. The milk sugar (lactose) is in the whey, so as it loses whey, it loses carbs. Cheese makers drain off whey to make cheese, which is why the harder cheeses have fewer carbs (essentially zero) than soft cheese and cottage cheese.

But among Greek yogurts, there's a wide range in carb contents, so read the labels and get the one with the fewest per cup. Between 5 grams and 9 grams is good; over 15 grams is too much. Always go for plain—anything added means more carbs.

You'll notice that craters in the tub of yogurt fill with liquid whey. Dump it out. The whey is sour and has lactose (milk sugar)—double whammy there—so get rid of it and the yogurt will be milder for it.

Full-fat yogurt tastes better, is richer than low-fat and nonfat yogurts, and on a super low-carb program, it'll fill you up without making you fat from the extra calories. If you're used to fruit-flavored, still buy it plain, but add a few berries and/or a little xylitol or stevia.

33 Booze trumps junk

If you were concerned about calories, you'd have to give up the empty ones from alcohol, but on a low-carb diet that doesn't count calories, as long as your total carbs are low enough, it doesn't matter where they come from.

The goal is to limit carbs to whatever quantity your body can tolerate while still burning fat for fuel, and maintaining a state of ketosis often enough to lose weight and be healthy—and that depends on your insulin sensitivity. If you get fat easily, you may have to limit yourself to 20 grams of carbohydrates per day; if you don't, you can probably eat 50 grams of carbs per day. This is good news for booze fans! Spirits are the lowest in carbs, beer is the highest, and always skip the mixers if they're sweetened.

Essentially zero carbs:
Whiskey, gin, rum, tequila, Scotch, vodka—as long as they're unsweetened and not mixed with sugared soda.

Some white wines are lower in carbs than others, and I'm listing only the lowest. Red wine is generally lower in carbs than white, so there is more variety. All wine servings are for a 5-ounce glass (there are five servings in a standard-sized bottle):

White:
Riesling: 6 grams
Champagne, sparkling wine: 3 grams

Red:
Burgundy: 6 grams
Claret, zinfandel: 5 grams

Chianti, Syrah, Petite Sirah, Merlot, Cabernet Sauvignon, Pinot Noir: 4 grams

Beer, per 12-ounce can or bottle:
most light beers: 3 to 9 grams
most regular beers: 12 to 15 grams

These cocktails have fewer than 5 grams each:
Tom Collins, highball, martini, gimlet, Gibson, sloe gin fizz, Manhattan, bloody Mary, Rob Roy

The danger of drinking alcohol while changing the way you eat is that it can lower your junk-food inhibitions and then all hell can break loose. But if being able to have wine with dinner is the difference between trying this way of eating and not, then cheers.

34 Going low-carb without going no-chocolate

I don't waste my daily carb allowance on bread and fruit; I spend it on chocolate. It's a good way to go as long as you're selective. Most of the good chocolate comes in a 100-gram (3.5-ounce) dark chocolate bar that measures roughly 3½ inches by 6 inches. You can buy them at Target, Trader Joe's, Whole Foods, airport shops—pretty much everywhere sophisticated adult candy is sold. The carb and sugar content is listed on the label for all to see, so read it. If a 100-gram bar has fewer than 12 grams of sugar (the digestible carbohydrates), it's not bad. If it has fewer than 7 grams, gobble it up.

If you're used to Hershey's chocolate bars, you won't immediately like cocoa content of more than 50 percent, but start at 50 and work your way to 85 and stop there. Ninety is no good. Once you can handle 85 percent—and you've given up grains and fruit—you can probably eat a whole bar a day and still be a fat burner in the best shape of your life. An even better, but more expensive, alternative is stevia-sweetened chocolate. Lily's is one brand; it's sweetened with erythritol and stevia, because pure stevia is too bitter for most palates. A 100-gram stevia-sweetened Lily's bar has less than 2 grams of sugar.

Steer clear of maltitol-sweetened chocolate. Maltitol triggers a glucose response, which defeats the purpose, and it can make your stomach upset. The best chocolate solution of all is to make your own. It costs a lot less, tastes better, fills you up with healthy fat, and doesn't jack up your blood sugar. See the Recipes section (page 206).

35 Quickie guide to fake sugars (which are not really fake)

As you know, among the most evil things you can put into your body is sugar. Natural or not, it's bad for you. Fake sugar is a different story. It's not health-boosting or actually beneficial by itself, but if you need some sweetness, this is where to turn.

Your first choice should be stevia, which comes from the stevia plant. It's known for its bitter aftertaste, but you can build up a tolerance for it. It comes in powder or liquid form, and in a range of flavors. There is no spike in glucose or insulin from stevia, so it's safer than a peach or a potato. Stevia scholars claim it's 300 times as sweet as sugar, but you'll need to use more than 1⁄300th as much stevia as you would sugar to get the same sweetness. Start with half a teaspoon in a cup of Greek yogurt, and see how it goes. You can also bake with it. Even better (less bitter) is NuStevia, a blend of stevia and maltodextrine, a carbohydrate. I use it when I make chocolate for people who expect all chocolate to taste like a candy bar.

Erythritol, despite its scary name, is another sweetener that's OK. It occurs naturally in some fruits, and like stevia, it doesn't jack up your blood sugar. It's about 60 percent as sweet as real sugar. You know that cooling sweetness of some sugarless gums and candy? That's erythritol. You can buy it online under that name in powders or granules for less than $10 a pound.

Xylitol is another favorite among health-conscious low-carbers. Like erythritol, it has a scary name, but it is found in some natural foods, and your body makes small amounts of it. It doesn't raise your blood sugar, so it's a perfectly good sweetener, but not a main course.

36 Eight foods to avoid at all costs

- **GRAINS**: Whole grains, refined grains, any grains. No bread, no pasta, no cereal, and no hidden grains. Grains make you fat by jacking up your blood sugar and insulin, preventing fat burning, and promoting fat storage. Nix them all forever.
- **SUGARS**: Sodas, jams, jellies, high-fructose corn syrup, and syrups of any kind. Foodmakers sneak sugar into salad dressings, marinades, sauces, and other condiments. I allow some sugar in my ketchup, but not high-fructose corn syrup. I've learned to like mustard on burgers, but I still sneak a small squirt of the red stuff. You can find Paleo ketchup online. Kids raised on Heinz won't love it, but it's OK.
- **FRUIT JUICE**: It's concentrated fructose, the most fat-producing sugar of them all. From a fattening point of view, you may as well drink a homemade mix of table sugar and water with artificial flavor and color.
- **SPORTS DRINKS AND ENERGY BARS**: They're devil-in-disguise foods, worse than soda and donuts, because at least soda and donuts don't trick you. Gatorade and a PowerBar? Fat and diabetic ex-athlete.
- **POTATOES**: Bereft of most nutrients except potassium, they are way too starchy for human health. If you're serious about health, regard all potatoes—even those presented like healthy, whole gems—like fast-food French fries.

- **CORN**: Super high in sugar, today's corn is a food created in labs to make it taste like candy. Just a little processing and that sugar-sweet corn on the cob in the produce section becomes the high-fructose corn syrup we've all been warned against.
- **WHITE RICE**: If it were merely worthless filler, that'd be one thing; but it's harmful filler, and cultures that eat a lot of it are alive in spite of it, not because of it. Don't eat white rice, and while you're at it, don't eat brown rice, either. It's 98 percent as bad for you.
- **HYDROGENATED OR PARTIALLY HYDROGENATED OILS**: These are trans fats, the most justifiably vilified of all "foodstuffs." Anything with this on the ingredients label is a no-go. These processed oils are everywhere, so read the labels. They are in most packaged baked goods, most supermarket sauces and dressings, cookies, bread, you name it.

37 Eleven foods to eat with gusto

"Eat with gusto" doesn't mean wolfing down so much food that you feel sick. When you're a fat burner, you won't want to eat as much, so stop when you're full—or slightly before. And always, for any food you eat—including the ones on this list—read labels and avoid bad ingredients. This is especially important if it's a prepared or canned food. Is there soybean oil in the tuna, or high-fructose corn syrup in the ketchup? Reading labels isn't about being fussy, it's about not being taken advantage of by companies that are making a buck off you while misleading you. The food on this list should be your everyday fare.

- **YOUNG, OILY FISH** like salmon, mackerel, and sardines: Young is good, because fish living in mercury-poisoned oceans accumulate mercury as they age and eat other contaminated fish. If you have a fishmonger near you, ask him to show you the young fish. Fish fat is especially good for you because it's high in omega-3 fatty acids, and fish has good protein and no carbs. Eat the skin if it's there—it's the fattiest part and the best tasting. Crisp-but-still-chewy salmon skin is my number one delicacy. When you buy salmon, get it with the skin on.
- **LEAVES:** The darker ones are more nutritious but also tend to taste stronger, so if you can't handle that, just go lighter. Their biggest contribution isn't their nutrition (we don't thoroughly digest cellulose-bound nutrients), but their relative harmlessness, visual appeal, and texture. Leaves, for

the most part, pass through and do little to no harm. It may seem like faint praise, but nobody ever becomes fat and unhealthy on them, and not many modern foods can claim that.

- **MAMMALS AND BIRDS:** Eat grass-fed, free-range, local, organic, and pesticide-free meat when possible, and that's fairly easy if you live near big cities or on a farm. Organ meats are especially nutrient-dense. Liver is off the charts in nutrition, but liver from grass-fed cows is hard to come by. So focus on meat from good farms, not factory farms.
- **COCONUT:** Especially coconut oil. It's low in omega-6 fatty acids, it's the best source of medium-chain triglycerides, which are readily available as fuel. Best of all, it's not stored as fat; it'll keep you in ketosis if you're already there. Every decent grocery store has it.
- **EGGS:** Free-range chickens are all over the place now, so there's no need to eat eggs laid by chickens that have spent their entire lives in a chicken-sized box with a lightbulb over it. Egg whites are all protein; the yolks are protein and fat. There are no carbs in eggs, so eat up. By the way, you'd think that a "free-range" chicken gets to roam around freely on the land, but there are no legal requirements, so a free-range chicken may get no more than its share of space in the chicken barn. Ethical egg shopping may mean that every now and then you buy the $5- to-$8-a-dozen eggs at the farmers' market. That's still a bargain, considering all you can get out of an egg.
- **OLIVE AND MACADAMIA OILS:** These are the best salad oils. Olive tastes better, but macadamia has fewer omega-6 fats. Try combining them.

- **MUSHROOMS:** Not being plants, they lack cellulose, so they're more digestible, but they're high in carb-free potassium (unlike potatoes or bananas).
- **BERRIES:** Strawberries, blueberries, blackberries, raspberries, huckleberries, boysenberries, gooseberries—compared to other fruits, they're low in carbs and rich in antioxidants. Eat them by the berry, not the mouthful.
- **BELL PEPPERS:** The darker the better. They're one of the few crunchy foods that's low in carbs and high in nutrients. How extractable those cellulose-bound nutrients are is not fully determined, but on a low-carb diet you'll eat them mainly as colorful crunch and tasty filler—which there's precious little of in the low-carb world. So go to town on peppers with no concerns of weight gain or diabetes.
- **AVOCADOS:** Fatty with good fat, filling, low carb, and they have minimal influence on blood sugar. And that's pretty much all that matters around here.
- **CHEESE:** It's good for you, assuming you can handle dairy. Even lactose-intolerant people can generally eat hard cheese, because the lactose was removed when the whey was drained. And the harder the cheese, the less whey, the less lactose, the less gas.

38 If you can afford this book, you can afford good food

The U.S. Department of Agriculture has said that it costs about $12.50 to feed a human body for a day. But if you're gainfully employed, aren't living hand-to-mouth, and now and then you eat in a restaurant, you probably spend more than that.

The eating plan I suggest—mostly fat, some protein, and as few carbs as you can manage—is inexpensive even when you buy good meat, mainly because when you get used to eating this way, you eat way less. Just as important, you *want* less, because you don't eat constantly. This is one of those states of being (along with not being ravenous when 5 hours have passed since you last ate, not waking up in the morning famished, and not having to take energy bars and drinks and snacks on a long bike ride) that seems impossible before you start burning fat, but becomes the normal state of affairs when you are. It's obviously cheaper to eat smaller amounts of food that keep you full than to gorge three times a day and graze in between, as sugar-burners on high-carb diets do.

Coming up are a couple of eating scenarios and their costs. Keep in mind that these sample menus work only after your body has adapted to low-carb eating—after about a week or two of drastically reducing carbs. As for the cost estimates that follow: They will vary, depending on whether you buy organic out or prepare factory-farmed at home, but you can hit that dollar figure with a reasonable effort and conscience.

SCENARIO NO. 1

BREAKFAST: Two to five tablespoons of butter or cream in your tea or coffee. You can make coffee at home for less than a buck, but let's round up: $1.00.

MIDMORNING SNACK: Two ounces of cheese ($1.50 for cheese that costs $12 per pound, which gives you lots of options), two ounces of salami ($3 for artisanal salami at $24 per pound): $4.50.

LATE LUNCH: Most of a can of wild salmon: $3.00.

DINNER: A four-ounce hamburger patty ($2—you can find grass-fed chuck for $8 per pound), one bunch of chard ($2, organic), and a small bowl of plain Greek yogurt with a few macadamia nuts ($1.50) = $5.50.

DAY'S TOTAL: $14.00.

SCENARIO NO. 2

BREAKFAST: Home-cooked omelet made with four eggs, two ounces of shredded cheese, and five strips of bacon (no nitrates): $6.00.

Tea or coffee: $1.00.

After this, you won't be hungry until 2:30 p.m.

LUNCH: 1 cup full-fat, plain Greek yogurt and an ounce of cheese. Go, Dairy! If you're lactose intolerant, sub a can of sardines for the yogurt: $3.00.

DINNER: Greek salad, village style (no lettuce—just cukes, tomatoes, onions, green or red peppers, olives, feta), one hard-boiled egg, and either 2 ounces of canned sardines or the meat of your choice; olive oil and vinegar dressing: $7.00.

DAY'S TOTAL: $17.00.

39 Viva canned fish!

Meat can be expensive, but on a high-fat diet, you aren't as hungry, so you don't eat as much, and since you aren't wasting money on bread, pasta, cereal, fruit, soda, and juices, you have money to spare for the wild and grass-fed meats that might have been beyond your budget before.

But even so, I'm a huge fan of cheap canned sardines, herring, and salmon. Sometimes I think stuffing fish into a can makes it taste better—maybe it's the vacuum-packing or months of contact with metal. Whatever it is, it's good and it's a bargain. Three dollars' worth of canned fish—ideally with the bones in and the skin on—is good hot, cold, or at room temperature; plain or mixed into salads, or Greek yogurt and macadamias, or omelets. I always think that if my life goes south and I go hobo, I'd do fine on less than $8 a day, as long as I could get canned fish.

Advice from a connoisseur: Brands vary tremendously in size, texture, firmness, and taste, so don't give up if you get a can of nasty on your first try. It's hard to go wrong with the Brunswick brand, and Trader Joe's smoked sardines and canned red salmon are my personal favorites, but there are more good ones than bad ones. Most of the canners have the formula down.

EXERCISE BASICS

The multibillion-dollar exercise industry counts on you to think of exercise as fun, but it's a trick. The most efficient, effective exercise is unpleasant, uncomfortable, and a relief to be done with. For your muscles to get stronger, they need to burn and you need to gasp, and it won't happen while you're reading a magazine or following your favorite tunes while on a treadmill. Easy exercise helps rehab patients become mobile again; it won't shape up an already mobile body.

The good news is that effective exercise takes no more than a few minutes a day, five days a week. You can still ride your bike, go skiing, surf, hike, swim, or even jog, but do them for fun instead of relying on them for exercise. And if they're not fun, don't bother. Consider this: The point of exercise is to make life easier and more fun and to make you more injury-resistant. To do that, you have to suffer a little. Not a lot, but definitely a little. It's kind of like an inoculation: effective, but not thrilling.

40 Don't jog

Humans have bigger brains than wild animals, and when it comes to exercise, that may be part of the problem: We combine facts and falsehoods in ways that animals can't, and come up with crazy ideas about exercise. There's no animal equivalent to the human jog, and before the moon landing, jogging was a fairly freakish behavior, even for us. Then in 1968, Kenneth Cooper's bestselling book *Aerobics* triggered the overexercising boom, and all we've gotten is more tired, injured, and fatter. Watch any public half or full marathon, and you'll see desperate people suffering long hours of ineffective, even dangerous, exercise.

We're so used to the idea of suffering being productive—studying for a test, scrubbing road rash, swallowing foul-tasting medicine—that even when it's not healthy, we think it is. Jogging feels healthy because it's dreadful, but it's the kind of dreadful that's counterproductive. Your body responds to too much running by releasing cortisol, a stress hormone. Cortisol triggers a process called gluconeogenesis, in which your muscles (made up of protein) break down into glucose. A lifestyle that includes hours of running every week can grind down your muscle, which causes the gaunt, wiry look of so many world-class marathon runners. The healthiest and arguably best-looking bodies in the sports world belong to sprinters, gymnasts, rock climbers, and dancers. They may have good genetics, but it is short, intense, straining, gasp-inducing exercise that shapes their bodies. They don't jog.

Jogging doesn't build strength or fitness—it just trains muscles to tolerate more jogging, and in the real world that's close to useless. You don't jog to a bus that's about to take off, or jog away from bad guys who are chasing you on foot. You *sprint*. Nobody ever jogged for a touchdown, or down the basketball court on a fast break, or across the tennis court to return a shot.

Jogging's reputation for being healthy doesn't jibe with reality. Do it if it's the way you like to wind down or relax, but don't do it for your physical health.

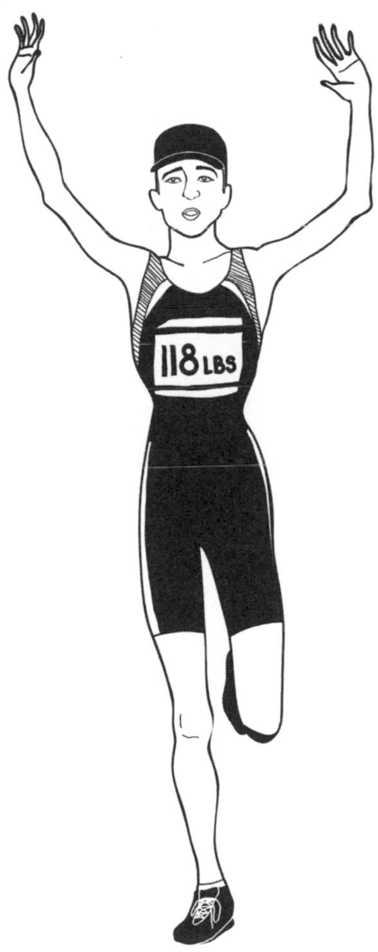

41 What kind of exercise works best?

Short, intense exercise that makes your muscles burn and makes you gasp for more air to supply the burning muscles with oxygen. It has to be hard. If you can talk or watch TV or maintain the effort level for more than 5 minutes, it's too easy. If you want maximum return on your exercising minutes—so you can make it as short as possible—you need to work as hard as you can.

This idea is antithetical to the "exercise is fun" notion that drives the exercise industry, but let me be clear about this. Skiing, hiking, riding a bike, and surfing are fun, but the exercise is incidental to the fun. Fun is great, but it's an inefficient way to get fit. I'm not saying don't do it—that stuff can be the best part of your life. I'm just saying that when the goal is improved cardiovascularity, stronger muscles, and injury resistance, then short, superintense exercise works much better and much faster than play or recreation. Maximally efficient exercise is barely bearable, and not even close to fun.

Your efficient time exercising can be as short as 3 to 7 minutes a day. Seven minutes is only about 1⁄200th of your day. When you're finished, you won't feel wasted like you do after a long ride or run. You'll fully recover in a few minutes and have the rest of the day to work, play, travel, explore, study, read, have sex, ride your bike, hike, and walk the dog. Short, intense workouts make your fun exercise easier and leave more time for life.

42 If your workout requires special clothing, it's the wrong kind of workout

Workout clothing is half unnecessary, half scam. If you already own grippy shoes that flex, and loose or stretchy pants, you have plenty of workout clothing already. Anything that allows squats and jumping jacks is fine for a 3- to 7-minute workout. You'll be finished with your workout in the time it takes to change costume, and with the workouts so short, you won't sweat and stink up whatever you're wearing. The jeans you chop wood in, the T-shirt you would never wear in public, the linen slacks that are not too tight, the blouse that makes you look ten years older and 20 pounds heavier—they're all perfect. Shoes are easy, too: Wear flat or low-heeled shoes or sandals, nothing with raised heels that pitch you forward. Or go barefoot.

If a new workout wardrobe supercharges your motivation, then go to town—but spend twice as much on kettlebells.

43 If you eat sugar, you can't exercise off your fat

If you've spent years trying to work off your fat to no avail, here's a way. Understanding this will help you to stop trying to do something that is truly impossible and beating yourself up for failing at it.

Most doctors, nutritionists, and the government still say weight management is simply a matter of burning more calories than you eat. They're the Flat Earthers, the Continental Drifters, the Creationists of weight management. What they say—that eating less and exercising more is a sustainable way to lose weight—ignores the effects of insulin. Weight gain or loss is all *about* insulin. Any discussion of calories eaten versus calories burned must include insulin's role in determining whether you burn sugar or fat, and something called *homeostasis*.

Homeostasis is your body's way of balancing input and output, and keeping you alive without your having to think about it: shivering to stay warm or sweating to cool down. When shivering alone won't warm you up, your desire to stay comfortable makes you put on a coat; and when it's hot out, it makes you strip off layers. When your body needs help keeping you comfortable, homeostasis calls you to action.

In eating and exercising, homeostasis trumps willpower and determination. Consider this: There are 3,500 calories in a pound of fat, whether the fat comes from a salmon, a pig, a pile of soybeans, or your belly. An hour of strenuous exercise burns 700 to 900 calories, depending on how big you are and how much you're able to suffer. But let's use the 700-calorie figure for now, because it's an effort level most people can sustain if they're forced to suffer for an hour in a jog.

To lose 1 pound mathematically, you have to exercise (at 700 calories per hour) for 5 hours, while consuming zero calories. The problem is that exercise makes you hungry, and when you're burning glucose—because you've not yet trained your body to burn its own fat for energy—you won't be able to exercise for more than 2 or 3 hours without requiring more glucose—supplied by more carbs. For every 700 calories of carbs you eat, you have to exercise another hour to stay on track for the 3,500 calories you need to burn off a pound of fat. That extra hour of exercise, in turn, is another hour spent working up an appetite.

If you survive a 5- to 7-hour jog and burn up 3,500 calories, you'll be starving in a few hours and will eat them back on, because homeostasis insists on a balance of output and input. Willpower has nothing to do with it. Your body *will* get back those lost calories, and your long jog will have been for nothing.

So if you've been jogging for the sole purpose of burning calories, you now have a scientific basis for knocking it off. Exercise tones muscles and keeps the blood flowing, calms you down, flushes you out, maybe even jacks up your endorphins. It is a good thing for many reasons, but weight loss isn't one of them. So enjoy your hikes, walks, rows, bike rides, and swims without any regard for the calories they burn up.

44 When you're a fat-burner, you *will* exercise off fat

When your blood sugar and insulin are low enough, you'll burn fat for fuel. Exercise requires fuel and fat is the original fuel for it—before carbs took over and forced you to burn glucose. When you're a sugar-burner, you run out of fuel so quickly that you have to keep eating or drinking sugar to replace it. That's what sports drinks are—sugar, with a little salt, potassium, magnesium, phosphorus, and calcium. Most energy bars are fancy cookies and candy bars—more sugar that you have to replace soon after it's burned up.

But when you burn fat as fuel, you don't run out, so there's no need to refuel. Even if you're as skinny as a clothesline, you have enough body fat to fuel a few days of running. You won't drain your tank.

Don't take this to mean you have to exercise a lot to lose fat. When you're a fat-burner, you burn fat whether you exercise or not. You burn fat when you're reading a book, parallel-parking your car, walking your dog or cat, even sleeping. You'll lose more fat faster if you exercise, because exercise burns off glucose, so it reduces your circulating insulin. But as long as it's coming off, what's the rush? Play for fun, and burn fat while you're at it—since you can.

45 If you can't jog yourself skinny, why are the world's best distance runners skinny?

For the same reason pro basketball players are tall, pro football players are huge, and gymnasts are short. Athletes with certain body types—tall, stout, skinny, short-torsoed, big-boned, tiny-boned, light-as-a-feather—find success in sports that favor it. Sometimes the sport gets credit for shaping the body, but it really just hones the foundation you inherited from your parents. You can work hard and compensate for the wrong body type, as 5-foot, 3-inch professional basketball player Muggsy Bogues proved. But if success in a sport matters to you, it's easier to follow your body type and hone your skills in the sport that makes sense for it.

Another reason that world-class distance runners are so skinny is *gluconeogenesis*. That's when chronic distance training is fueled by glucose (carbs) and triggers an outpouring of cortisol, which causes your muscle (protein) to break down and form glucose for energy. This process of burning off muscles results in that wiry, emaciated look.

But there are plenty of runners and riders who remain stout despite the endless miles of training, because they're burning off some of the food they eat instead of their body fat. They're eating the high-carb sports foods that the industry tells them to eat in order to fuel their exercise.

46 When the goal is strength, high reps waste time

If you can do more than 15 reps of any lifting, pushing, pulling, strength-building exercise, the weight's too light. You need to burn deep in your muscles and make them scream for more oxygen. That's where "no pain, no gain" came from. It may sound like ancient dogma from the Cold War era, but it's valid. Not ligament-tearing pain, not tendon pain, not piercing joint or pulled-muscle pain, but muscles-burning-for-lack-of-oxygen pain.

To know what burning, muscle-building pain feels like, go into a deep squat, hold it for 5 seconds, then rise out of it slowly, taking 30 seconds to stand up all the way. The pain in your thighs is muscle-building burn.

The most effective way to make your muscles burn with any exercise is to either increase the weight so you get to the hard, grunting part of the lifting earlier in the rep set, or lift so slowly that the lactic acid (that's the burn) builds up.

One great way to get strong faster is to pick a weight (heavier!) or a speed (slower!) that stops you at 6 reps—but instead of lifting 6 times, lift 5. Avoiding the sixth rep reduces the micro muscle tears that you need to recover from when building muscle. If you're hell-bent on getting strong fast, you can repeat the exercise several times a week, with no need for recovery, and if you add this kind of workout to your regular ones, you'll be clearly, obviously, visibly stronger in a month.

47 Write your routine on a 3-by-5-inch card, then follow it

You don't need a cheerleader, coach, or personal trainer for a 5- to 7-minute workout, but you may need something to egg you on and keep you on track. So write your routine on an index card. Then you don't have to remember anything, and you can mentally (or actually) cross each set out as you complete it. Besides, if your workout is properly hard, you might not remember the order without a list.

Keep your completed lists around awhile: Date them and throw them in a shoe box or stick them on a spike. A few months later, you'll look at them en masse and you'll know you've done all that, and you're stronger now.

48 Make the most of a gym

If you've never lifted weights and want to start, but don't want to embarrass or hurt yourself, then OK—go to a gym and hire a personal trainer. Just don't get hooked on the trainer or on the machines. The machines have nothing to do with real-life weight lifting. When you lift a box of books or logs, or a cooler full of food and ice in one hand and some canvas chairs in the other as you walk to the beach, you engage all of your muscles trying to stay balanced, and you don't sit or lie down to do it. Real-life lifting and carrying require balance and all-body strength—your stomach muscles firing to keep you balanced while you're lifting a wiggly or uneven load. Racked weights allow some muscles to sleep while the others strain, and that doesn't train you for real-world work. Gyms need the machines, because if the floor was largely empty, with a few bars, balls, kettlebells, and other equipment you could buy yourself, you'd think twice about the monthly fees.

After a few weeks on the machines, train with free weights—barbells, dumbbells, and, if the gym is hip enough to have them, kettlebells. They're "free" in the sense that they're not on pulleys or moving in tracks defined by a machine, so you have to balance them as you lift, just as you do when lifting and carrying a cooler with one arm and beach chairs with the other. Balancing weight as you lift strengthens more muscles and simulates real-life weight lifting.

Once you've gained a little strength and familiarity with weights at the gym, thank your trainer, give him or her a big cash tip, and fly solo with even more effective and much shorter workouts. Use the floor to do balance ball or medicine ball push-ups. Do pull-ups, push-ups, sit-ups, and dips. Do burpees. If there's a pool, swim some. Use the exercise bikes or rowing machines to do Tabatas—20 seconds of full-blast effort followed by 10 seconds of rest, repeated 8 times (as described in The brutal Tabata, page 123). Use the dumbbells or kettle-bells, and do get-ups, presses, and squats. The "no weight machines" success of CrossFit gyms is spilling over to mainstream gyms, which now offer classes that emphasize intensity and variety without weight machines. There's plenty to do at a gym without the machinery.

49 Mixing work and play wrecks both

Exercise *can* be fun and play *can* be exercise, but if your 6-hour, 15-mile hike with 5,000 feet of elevation gain is fun only when it's over and you get to talk about it, then you're confusing pride or relief with fun. It's easy to do that.

It's far better to exercise efficiently during a concentrated 4-minute workout, and just relax and enjoy the bike ride. Then, if you're with slower riders, you can ride their pace and keep them company, instead of riding ahead to get your workout, and then waiting for them at the top of the climb. That just makes them feel bad for holding you back. In the old days, I used to do that sort of thing when I'd ride my bike or hike with my family and friends. If I rode with them, I'd think, "This is a bummer—I'm not getting a workout."

One of the points of losing weight and getting fit by cutting carbs and condensing your exercise into a few intense minutes is to turn what used to be hard drudgery into easier fun. Then, when you're riding alone, you can go farther or higher and see more in the same amount of time. And when you're with not-as-fit friends, you can go at a social pace and not feel like you're getting cheated out of a workout.

50 Don't cheat your muscles with momentum

It's hard to budge a car that's out of gas by pushing it, but once somebody else helps get it going, any credit hogger can chuckle and trot alongside, "helping" to push with a finger resting on the taillight. That's the power of momentum, and it cheats your muscles out of a workout. This is the easiest thing in the world to test. Take any exercise you can do, say, 5 at a relatively fast rate in less than 10 seconds: push-ups, body weight squats, climbing stairs. Now try completing the same number of reps in a minute. Next, stretch it to a minute and a half. Your muscles will burn and you probably won't make it. The burn is your muscles working without enough oxygen (anaerobically), and that's what builds muscles. Faster reps mean you're using too much momentum and not enough muscle, proof that the weight's too low.

51 Walking is a big part of the plan

The most beneficial exercises are at the extreme of the effort spectrum—easy movements and only slightly elevated heart rate and breathing at one end; sweaty, grunting, burning muscles and gasping for breath at the other. Habitual long and hard exercisers tend to think walking is a waste of time, but it's actually one of the best uses of time. It's the original human movement that separated us from the apes. It's not hard enough to build strength, but it's still one of the best because it keeps the blood flowing and heart pumping and muscles working at an all-day pace without any stress to your system. If your body is sore from too much the day before, walk. If you just don't feel like grunting, walk.

Your goal is a combination of short, grunty, muscle-burning exercises that you can do only for a few minutes, and then something easy—like walking, fun bike rides, or playing Marco Polo in a swimming pool. When you're exercising to get strong and improve your physical condition, stay out of the middle zone of "hard but sustainable." It's the exercise levels in the middle—sweating on the elliptical machine for 45 minutes, or a huffy-puffy hour-long jog—that you're best off avoiding. Do that kind of exercise to wind down or as a form of meditation, but not for its physical benefits.

52 Sit down at work or at home, but not both

Sitting down wrecks backs, weakens muscles through inactivity, and bogs down circulation. If you have a desk job, make a standing workstation out of boxes and plywood, or buy a prefabricated one for hundreds of dollars. Have a tall stool nearby for when you just have to sit down, but make standing, not sitting, your default working position.

A standing station is a good idea for zoning out in front of the television, too. You can probably find a podium at a tag sale and use it for books or newspapers or a laptop at home.

If I were rich and had the room, and if treadmills weren't so ugly, I'd have one so I could watch *The Big Bang Theory* and *Modern Family* while walking slowly. It wouldn't be for burning calories, but just to keep the blood flowing, the muscles lightly firing, and avoiding the back pains that come from sitting. I stand at work, sit at home, but not for more than 30 minutes at a stretch.

53 Stretch dynamically, not statically

The pain you feel behind your knee when you're trying to touch the floor is ligaments stretching beyond their comfort zone. Ligaments connect bones, and when they get too stretchy, they don't hold your joints in place as well, and you can get injured more easily. We humans overstretch, because we associate the pain with benefit. Animals never overstretch, because if something hurts, they stop. You've seen a dog or cat stretch when it gets up from a nap. It's a 3-second stretch, if that. If it lasted a minute, you'd call the vet in a panic. Your morning stretch can be 30 seconds, but a bit less is fine, too. Try a deep squat, staying down there and twisting; or hang from a pole to stretch your spine; or get inspired by your dog and do the downward dog yoga pose.

Stretching before a specific workout is another thing. There are two kinds of preworkout stretching: static and dynamic. Static is the bad kind, the old kind from the Khrushchev era, where you stay more or less still, stretch one thing at a time, and try to push through the pain. It's standing flat-footed and stretching toward the floor, or sitting down with straight legs in front of you and trying to touch nose to knees. Oddly, static stretching is still popular among those who don't know, and stretching this way before exercising makes your muscles relax, which makes them less prepared for the impending exercise, and makes you more likely to get hurt doing it.

The good kind of stretching is dynamic stretching, where you run your muscles through the same workout you're warming up for, but a lighter version of it. A golfer or baseball player takes a few swings before stepping up; a sprinter high-knee jogs around the track and takes a few running starts before a 100-meter sprint. This is dynamic stretching—pumping blood to the muscles about to be worked.

Following are examples of dynamic stretching for the exercises in this book:

- Swing a kettlebell that's half the weight you'll use in your workout.
- Do a few slow burpees or squats before your burpee or squat routine.
- Press a light weight a few times before pressing a heavy one.
- Do stretchy-band-assisted pull-ups or high-hand push-ups before real ones.

54 Don't make a big production of warming down

Warming down is another of those "human-only" practices that catch on only because somebody can make what sounds like a convincing argument, despite its total lack of validity. The warm-downers say to taper off your exercise gradually, rather than just stopping and catching your breath. But after a cheetah catches and kills the zebra, he doesn't lope lightly in circles around dinner. Migrating birds and spawning salmon don't fly and swim around aimlessly once they've reached their spots. Only modern, exercising humans do it.

The exercises that follow don't require warm-downs. Just walk around for 5 seconds, flop on the floor or a bench while your heart rate and breathing get back in sync, then get back to your real life.

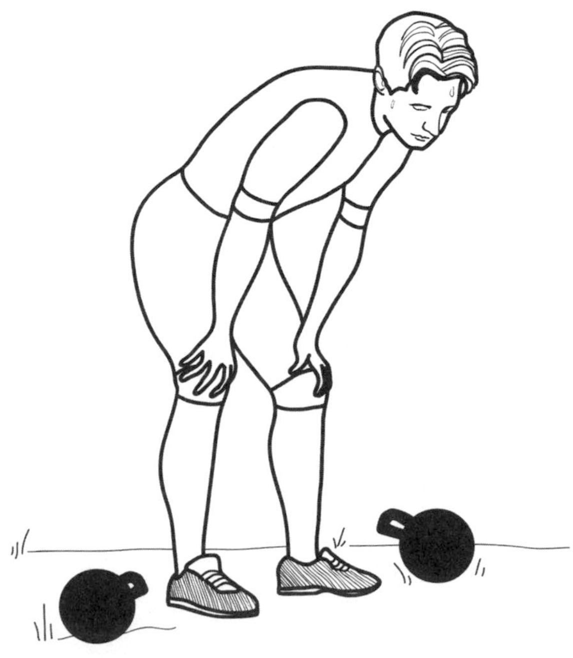

EXERCISE PARTICULARS

The exercises that follow fall into two types: body weight and kettlebells. Body weight exercises don't require special equipment and you can do them anywhere—indoors or out.

The kettlebell exercises require kettlebells, which start at about $30, take up almost zero floor space, and never wear out. For the cost of a half a year's gym membership, you can get half a dozen kettlebells that'll last you to your grave, at which point you can pass them on to your heirs.

These tough-love exercises are a starting point for your own made-up, burning-and-gasping whole-body exercises, or they can be all you do. Either way, you're covered.

55 Russian push-ups

You know the basic push-up. The Russian version looks 98 percent the same, but is 700 percent harder, and the difference is elbow placement and speed. In a Russian, your elbows are just outside your ribs, and you push up in 2 to 4 seconds, let yourself down in 2 to 4 seconds, hold it there for a second, and repeat until you can't anymore. Don't be bummed if you find you can do only one or two.

Keeping your elbows close to your ribs loads the work onto your triceps (back of your upper arm), rather than thrusting so much onto your pectorals (chest muscles); and going slowly prevents you from using speed and momentum to cheat yourself out of a real workout. 1 2

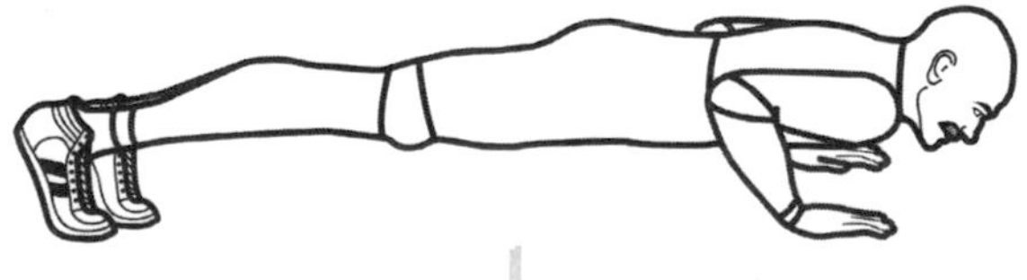

If you can't do them slowly at first, speed up, or try American push-ups, with your elbows sticking out. If you still can't do any, pivot off your knees, not your feet—in the old days, this was known all over the country as a girl's push-up, because they were standard form for girls in school physical fitness tests; this is how girls were expected to do push-ups. If the name bothers you, try this: Stand about 4 feet away from a wall or a table, and put your hands flat on the surface with your elbows at your sides. Push yourself away from the surface. It's easier because you're pushing up less weight, but using the same Russian form—elbows at your sides, at shoulder height, hands. The higher your hands and the faster you push up, the easier it is. After a month or so of four-day-a-week Russian wall or table push-ups and progressively lowering your hands, you'll be doing real Russians on the floor.

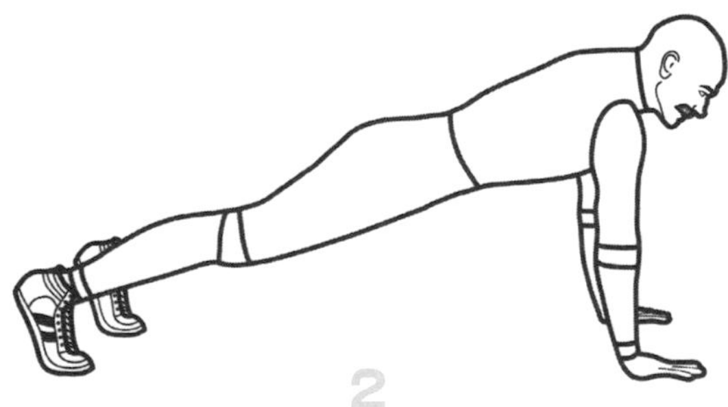

56 Janda sit-ups

The standard sit-up, where you lock your feet under a sofa or somebody holds them down, are easy because they use your hip flexors, not just your abs. But they also stress your spine and can cause lower back pain or make it worse. Janda sit-ups are better in all ways. They rely entirely on your stomach muscles (exactly what you want), and they don't stress your back. The downside is that you probably can't do one right now—I bet fewer than 1 adult in 500 can. They're hard to like, but they give you a hard stomach, and you can work up to one. When you can do one, you're a month away from ten. There's no reason to ever do more than ten of these.

Lie on your back on the floor, knees bent, the soles of your feet on the floor, your arms crossed in front of your chest. 1

Have somebody block your heels with their hands.

Keep your feet flat and your knees bent, then sit up slowly, clenching your butt and flexing your hamstrings, as though you're trying to pull your heels toward your butt. 2 With your butt and hamstrings (backs of your thighs) flexed, your abdominals will do all the work, and your lower back won't suffer.

There are several ways to work toward getting all the way up. Ten of these twice a week will give you the hardest abs of your life.

- Downhill sit-ups: Find a lawn with a slight slope. Sit with your legs down the hill so your head is higher than your feet. Try the above exercise again. This is easier than a level-floor Janda, but uses the same muscles. Once you can do 10 downhill Jandas, find

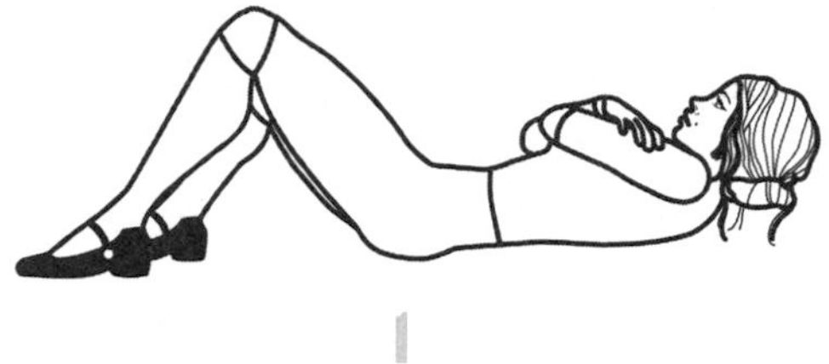

1

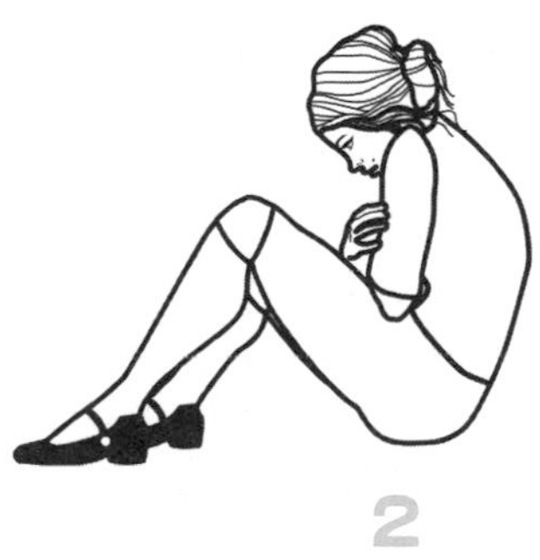

2

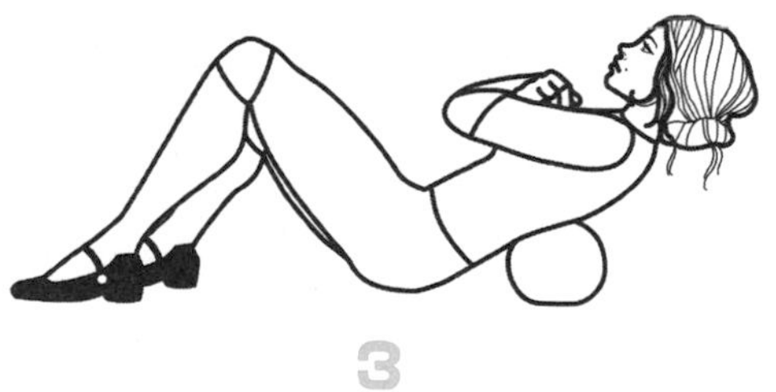

3

a lower slope and work up to 10 again. Keep making your way to a flat surface until you're doing a floor Janda.

- Halfway sit-ups: Start halfway up and stop halfway down. Stack pillows or an exercise ball behind you to limit how far you can lean back. 3 Start with your knees bent and your heels blocked. Let yourself down just far enough that you can sit back up. Do 10 of these well before lowering the cushion, increasing the range. Over time, lower the cushion height until you're doing real Janda sit-ups.
- Raised torso sit-ups: Lie down on a raised bed with your feet on the floor. The "raised bed" isn't something you find at the gym store, but with some scrounging and creativity you can make a 4- to 6-inch-high cot-width platform long enough to support your body from butt to head while your feet are flat on the floor. Gradually lower the platform until you can do Jandas on a level floor.
- Momentum sit-ups: Cheat by using momentum—at first. Throw your arms into it, letting them create the momentum you need to sit up. After enough cheating successes, gradually reduce the cheating until you can do them with folded arms.

57 Push-ups with benches, chairs, and balls

Push-ups are the easiest of the body-weight calisthenics because you're not lifting your whole body weight. That makes them ideal for a starter exercise. Once you can do twenty-five, make them harder and more beneficial for your new strength. Here are some different push-ups:

- High-feet push-up: Elevate your feet on a bench or sofa, hands on the floor. The higher your feet, the harder the push-up.
- Basketball push-up: Put one hand on a basketball, the other on the floor. Roll the ball from hand to hand at the top of every push-up. When you stagger your hand height, the lower hand's arm works harder, so alternating arms will keep your muscle-building symmetrical.
- Balance-ball push-up: Put your feet on one of those big balance balls, toes down. Bigger balls = higher feet = harder push-ups. Combining higher feet with the need to balance makes these the hardest push-ups yet. Adding a basketball under one of your hands makes them even harder.

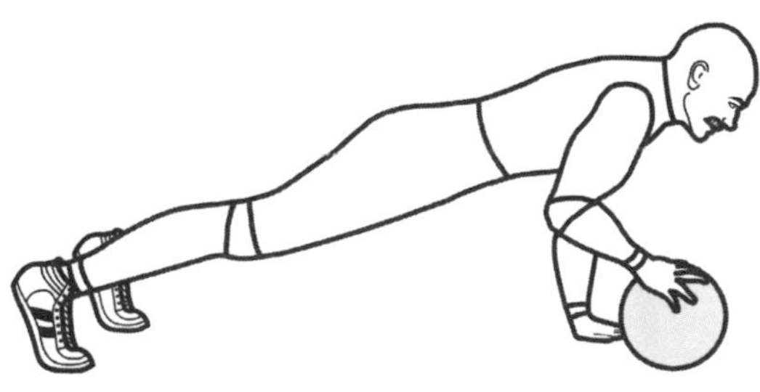

58 Pull up like a monkey

When you're hanging on the bar unable to pull yourself even halfway up, you think it's impossible to actually pull yourself up, ever. But there are ways to work up to it, and once you can do one, another two will take you about ten days. Keep it up and you'll be doing 10 within three months.

The best way to work up to a pull-up is to cheat with resistance bands—giant rubber bands color-coded by strength and available at specialty exercise-gadget supply stores. Loop one over the bar, stick your feet in the lower loop to stretch it out, and then as it rebounds to its relaxed length, it lifts you up to the bar like an invisible grandpa hoisting you up so you can see over the fence. Use a band that allows you to do 5 or 6 of these assisted pull-ups. As you get stronger, use lighter bands. After you've decreased the band strength three or four times, you won't need them anymore.

But let's say you're too broke to buy the bands, or are just philosophically opposed to them. You can still work up to a pull-up with let-downs, sometimes known as negative pull-ups. They're not quite as effective, but they'll work. Use a stool to get your head above the pull-up bar to chin height, then step off the stool and hold yourself there for a second or two before letting yourself down slowly. Rest a minute or two and repeat 6 or 7 times. Then give your muscles a day to recover and rebuild, and do it again.

Once let-downs are easy enough, start from the same position—chin above bar—and let yourself down 1 inch, then pull back up, repeatedly. Over several weeks, add inches to the drop and pull-up until you can do a whole one.

If you can do 20 pull-ups, you're doing them too fast. Go slower and burn your muscles longer with fewer reps. A 5- to 10-second pull-up may not look impressive, but it builds strength fast. It's muscle-burning time, not quantity and rapidity, that counts.

Injury prevention tip: Start your pull-up with your shoulders squared away from your ears, and when you're hanging from the bar, you obviously don't want to let your weight pull your shoulders out of their sockets, and you don't want to stress your arm tendons. To avoid that, do not straighten your arms entirely. While you are hanging, pull your shoulders downward, away from your ears. You can think of this as "reverse shrugging." Pulling up from completely straight arms stresses tendons, so go down 95 percent, but not 100 percent.

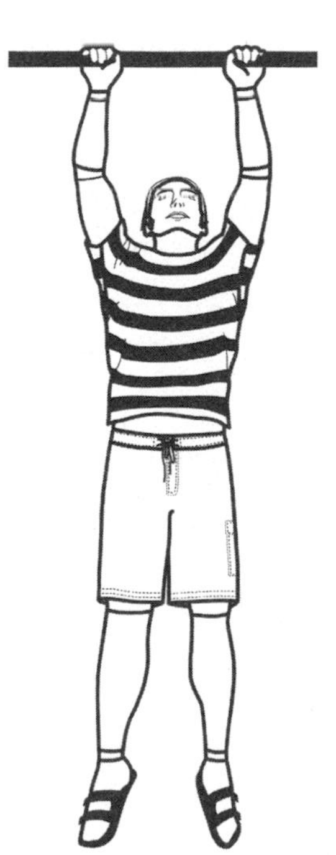

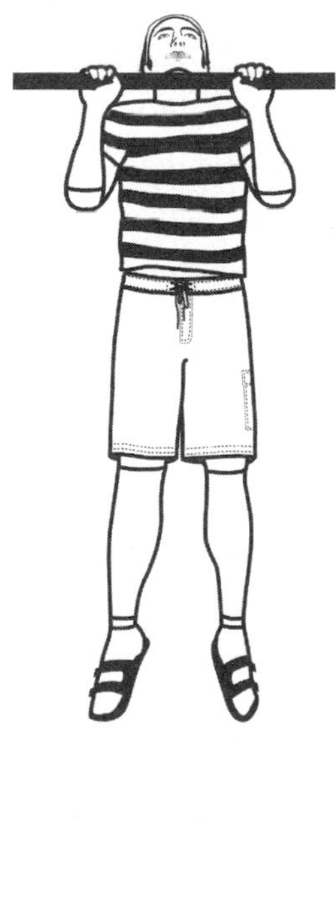

59 Dips

A lot of people can wiggle out a push-up or swing and kick out a pull-up or two, but unassisted dips are in their own league. If you climb trees or rocks or have to get over a fence now and then, you'll have an easier time of it if you've done your dips. As a bonus, dips build rounded, muscled deltoids (shoulder muscles).

In the basic dip, you grab parallel bars with your hands about 20 to 24 inches apart (wider than your shoulders, at least). Jump or use a stool to get yourself to the top position, with your feet off the ground and your arms straight. 1 Then bend your elbows outward (as opposed to keeping them close to your ribs) to lower yourself until the bottom of your ribs are near your hands. 2 Then push yourself up again. Sticking your elbows out helps protect your shoulders from injury.

There are two ways to work up to a dip—let-downs and jump-ups.

- Let-downs. Use a step to get into the top position—arms straight, feet aloft—then hold yourself there as long as you can. Once you can hold it for 15 seconds, you're strong enough to try lowering yourself. First lower yourself until your hands are outside your hips, and see if you can push yourself back up. Then lower to your waist and do the same. The maximum dip is when your hands are just outside your lower ribs, and it'll take three to six weeks of 5 minutes every other day, and when you work on the let-down and inch-up 10 minutes a week, you'll be there in a month.

- Jump-ups. Use a stool and push up with your legs to make it easier on your arms. This is cheating, but it's good cheating, and it gets around the challenge of rigging elastic bands above the dip station (assuming the dip station isn't directly beneath a pull-up bar). Gradually reduce the leg help until you can make it up with arms alone.

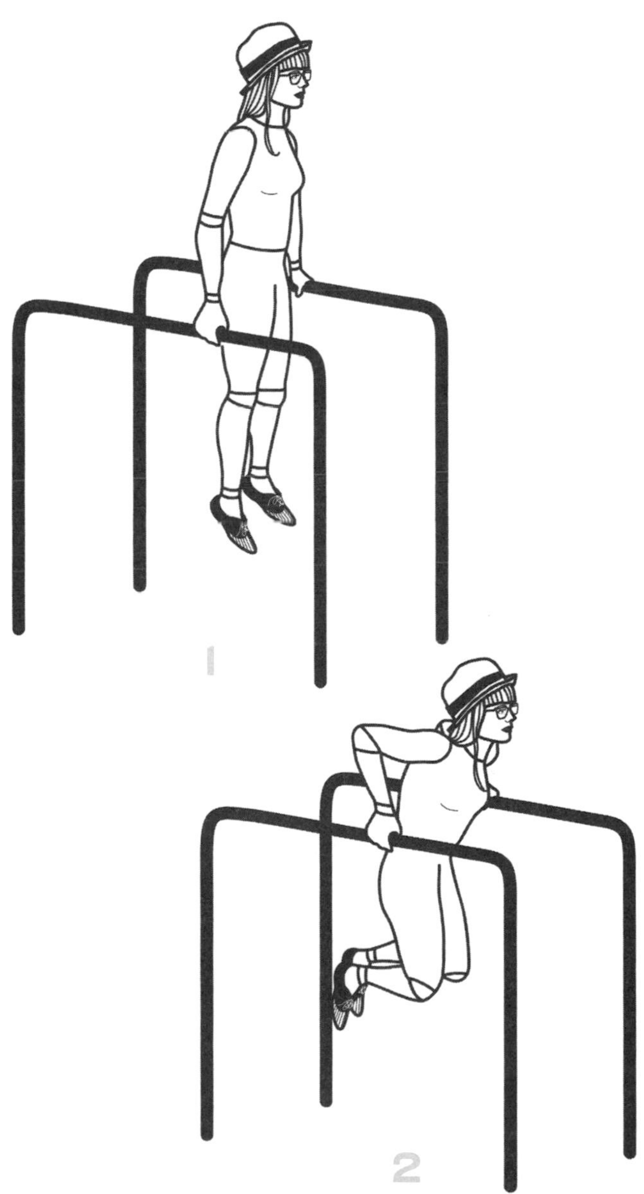

60 Crawl like a bug, but less efficiently

Crawling on your hands and feet (no knees allowed) is a slow, clumsy, awkward exercise; sometimes the break you need from an exercise program that's lung-taxing and form-demanding. It's not hard enough to make you gasp for breath or make your muscles burn, but it is hard enough to count as a legitimate workout and part of a bigger plan.

You can crawl anywhere, but I like to use a football field to make counting the distance easier. Here's how:

Start at one goal line and crawl on your hands and feet to the opposite one, or as close as you can get to it. If you collapse on the way, rest up for a minute and start again. Somehow, grunt and strain your way along the length of the field, or for 2 minutes, whichever comes first. Time counts, distance doesn't, so if 2 minutes brings you only to your own 25-yard line, that's fine.

With your first attempts at crawling, you'll think your technique is off, but it's not. You didn't evolve to crawl in this way, so it's just awkward. From an exercise point of view, that's a good thing. Trying to maintain your balance and move forward this way works your arms and the top of your thighs and every muscle in your core. Nothing relaxes, even for a second. When one side's foot and hand are in the air, your whole body tenses to maintain balance. Crawling is an odd exercise, but a good all-rounder.

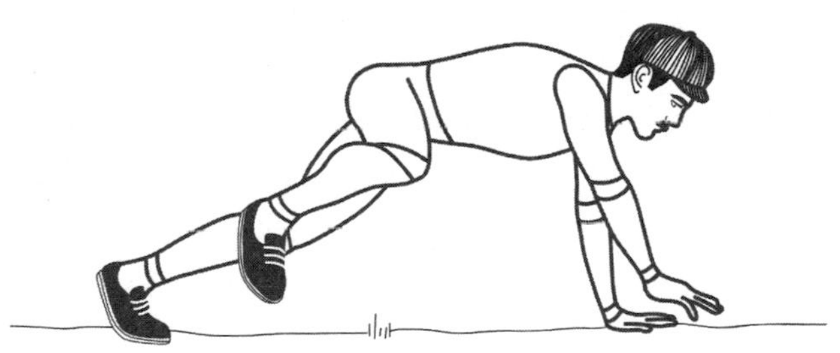

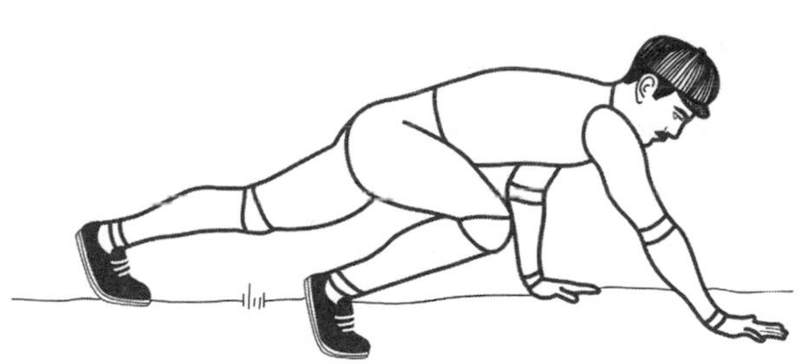

61 Squat right

Squats keep you strong when you're young, out of a wheelchair when you're old, and make carrying a load of books up three flights of stairs or getting out of a low car seat slightly easier. A proper squat prevents injuries and is a key part of a lot of the exercises in this book, so learn good form.

- Feet flat on the floor, slightly wider than your shoulders, toes pointed out a bit. Go barefoot or wear flat-soled shoes. 1
- Stand with your feet about 6 inches in front of a pole or wall. Try to maintain a consistent gap between your face and the wall or pole—as opposed to leaning forward and into it. Use your arms as counterweights—folded or sticking out straight in front of you (easier with a pole than a wall). 2
- Fold inward at the hips while your butt moves back, as if to sit on a stump behind you. Your knees will remain only slightly forward of your ankles, and your shins will be nearly vertical. 3
- Keep your back straight. Not straight up; just straight. It helps to look a little above your line of sight while keeping your head level.
- Inhale on the way down, exhale on the way up. Go down until you're almost sitting on the imaginary stump. You'll feel it in your thighs.

- Keep your weight on your heels or midfoot, not on the balls of your feet. You should be able to wiggle your toes or lift them up.
- Once down, hold for a second, then come up.

Once you have the form down, squat slowly to gain strength. One-second squats don't count; 5-second ones are much tougher; 15-second squats are killers. The burn you feel in your thighs makes them stronger.

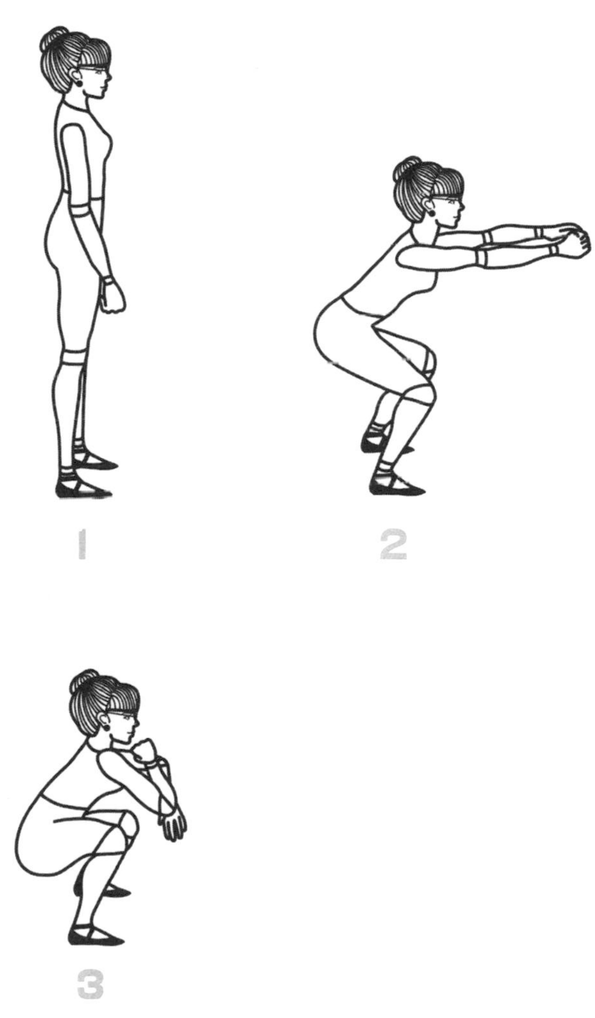

62 Jump like a kangaroo

From a standing start, drop to a deep squat. 1 Then rise and spring into a jump, pulling your knees as high as you can, trying to hit your chest. 2 You may not get them all the way up—I can't, either—but that's OK, because the benefit is in the effort, not the chest pummeling.

Kangaroos are entirely a leg exercise, so they're especially good when your arms and shoulders need a break. Start with 1, and work up to 10 in a row. Add these kangaroos into varied routines, or make a full routine of them—countdowns, Tabatas, Fibonacci, or if you're really tough, turn your burpee jump into a kangaroo.

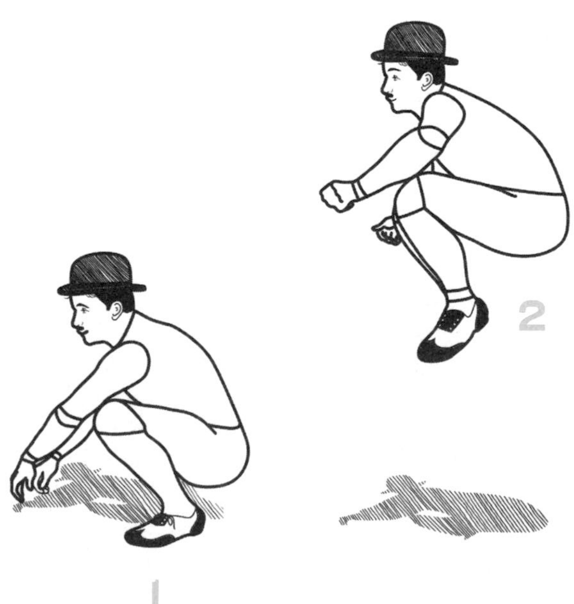

63 The amazing kettlebell

Kettlebells are cast-iron balls with handles, invented by Russians in the early 1700s. They were popular in the United States in the early 1900s, but over time, more gimmicky exercise devices took the lead. Then in 2001, a Russian guy—Pavel Tsatsouline (pronounced *sat-soo-leen*)—reintroduced them here, and what a great deed that was. Now you can buy kettlebells in many colors at any store that carries sports equipment. A kettlebell is the most effective all-body workout gizmo you can own, and since a kettlebell of any size takes up less floor space than a pair of shoes, six can be tucked away in a corner. Kettlebells are so effective that once you start using them, you'll think of your life as pre-kettlebell and post-kettlebell.

Russians measure kettlebells in *poods*. In America, kettlebells are marked in pounds or kilograms, sometimes both:

1 pood = 16 kilograms = 35 pounds

1.5 poods = 24 kilograms = 53 pounds

2 poods = 32 kilograms = 70 pounds

Common sizes range from 5 pounds up to 50-plus pounds, but specialty fitness stores stock them up to at least 70 pounds.

Start your kettlebell life with four bells. One should be superlight—maybe 5 pounds—to get the form down and to use when trying new moves. After learning the form, most women should get going with two 12-pounders and a 20, and most men with two 25-pounders and a 35. If there's any doubt, err on the light side.

Following are six kettlebell exercises that'll work all of your muscles. Three would probably do it, but I've included six for variety. There are lots of other kettlebell exercises, and once you know these you can smoothly transition to them if you like. But there's no real need, since these work every muscle you've got.

One last word here: Don't be intimidated or even inspired by the phenomenal and otherworldly kettlebell workouts you see on YouTube. Some people just like to show off under the guise of instruction. You can learn good form from them, but demonstrating to strangers how to do a Turkish get-up by using a 70-pound kettlebell is passive-aggressive boasting.

64 Kettlebell two-hand swing

If you had to limit yourself to one kettlebell exercise, this could be it. The two-hand swing is a workout for your legs, butt, lower back, arms, grip, shoulders, upper back, and heart, and it's the easiest to learn. But learn to squat first, because squatting is part of the two-hand swing.

Start with your feet on the floor, a bit wider than your shoulders, with a single kettlebell about 6 inches in front of your toes. 1

To pick up the bell, bend at the knees, stick your butt out, keep your back straight, and lift with both hands. 2

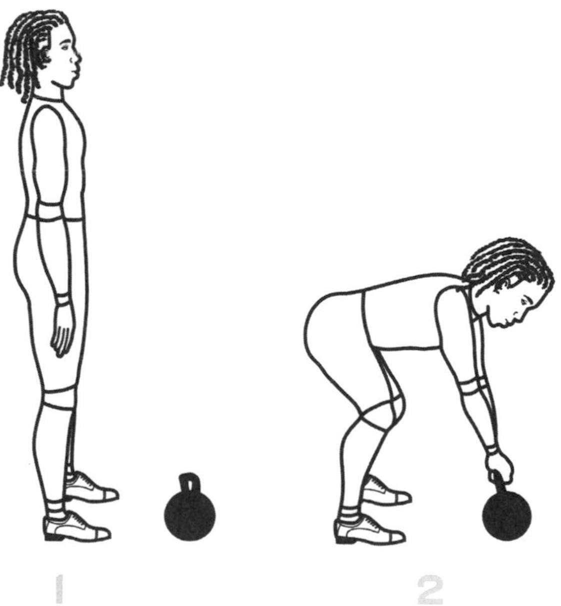

1 2

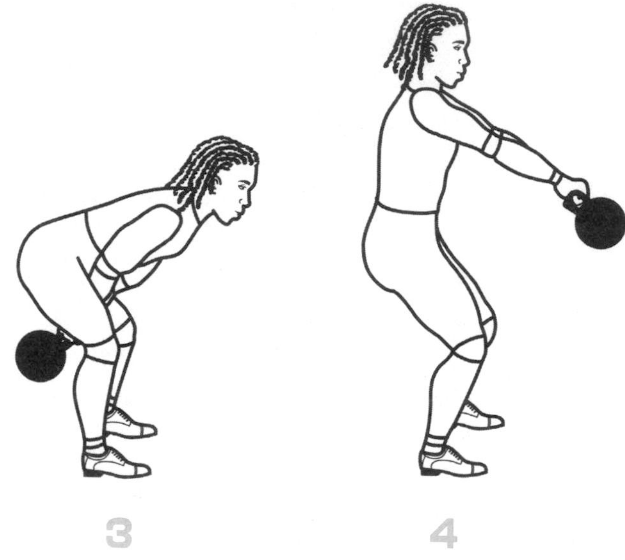

As the kettlebell clears the ground, it'll swing back between your legs. 3

As it swings forward, propel it upward with a mix of leg straightening, hip thrusting, and a little arm lifting. 4

The first upswing will probably go up to your belly height, but on the next forward swing, give it a little hip action, and it'll fly up as high as your chest. 5

Keep your back straight, your butt back, your shins vertical—good squat form. Weight your heels and look above the horizon to discourage bending your back. You'll naturally exhale on the downswing. When the bell is swinging, the handle should be in line with your forearms—vertical when your arms are down, horizontal when your arms are swinging up. If it droops below, you're not using enough hip oomph or the weight is too heavy. If the kettlebell flies high above your hands at the top of the swing, you can swing a heavier one. Heavier swing weights require deeper squats and more hip action to raise them above your eye level.

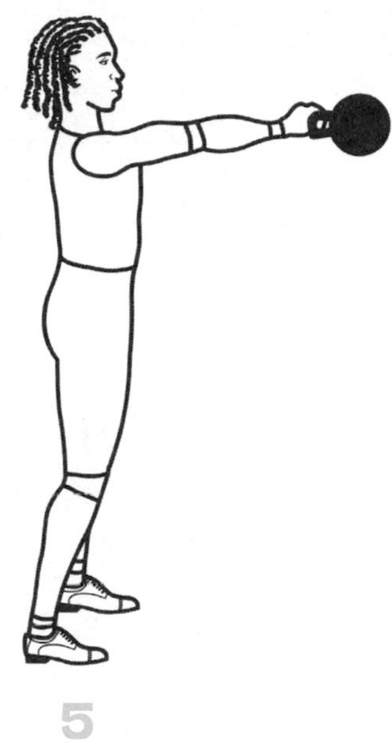

5

How many swings? Learn the form with 5 to 10 swings, and once you've got it, graduate to 15 or 20 in a set, then rest a minute and do it again. The next day you'll feel sore in your inner thighs, a reminder that you're exercising muscles that haven't had much action. Give it a rest for a few days before your next swing session, and after that, the pain won't return.

Start light (one-eighth to one-sixth of your body weight) and after 4 or 5 months of swinging for 2 minutes twice a week, you'll be swinging one-fourth of your body weight, and from there, it's a quick step up to one-third. I can't imagine the practical benefit of swinging more than, say, 40 percent of your body weight.

For a supereffective, supershort workout, two-hand swing a kettlebell for a minute and a half. Two variations follow.

- Instead of swinging a single kettlebell of, say, 35 pounds, try two of 15 pounds each; or a 15 in one hand, a 20 in the other. Mismatched kettlebells are harder, so it's more beneficial, and saves you the cost of a set of duplicate 25 pounders or whatever. Spread your legs an extra few inches and keep the handles parallel with the swing (aimed forward and backward).

- The one-hand swing. Start the swing in the same way as the two-hand swing, but use one hand, positioned in the center of the handle. When you pick up the bell and it swings between your legs, your free arm will swing behind you slightly, outside your legs. As the kettlebell goes up, the free arm goes along with it, and you switch hands at the top. Grab the handle a bit to the side to make more room for the incoming hand. I like two-handers for workouts, but it's good to learn the one-handers, too, because they're components of other kettlebell exercises.

65 Kettlebell squat

Get in good squat form (you learned it on page 100). Now add a kettlebell. Here are three ways to hold it:

- By the handle, ball on top and held high on your chest, elbows down.
- Easier: hanging straight down by the handle, like a two-hand swing grip. 1
- Like a kid lifting a bowling ball, with locked fingers underneath it.

Inhale on the way down, exhale on the way up. The goal is a deep, slow squat, to maximize the muscle-burn time. 2 Work up to it over a week or two, and if your knees are bad, do body-weight squats instead.

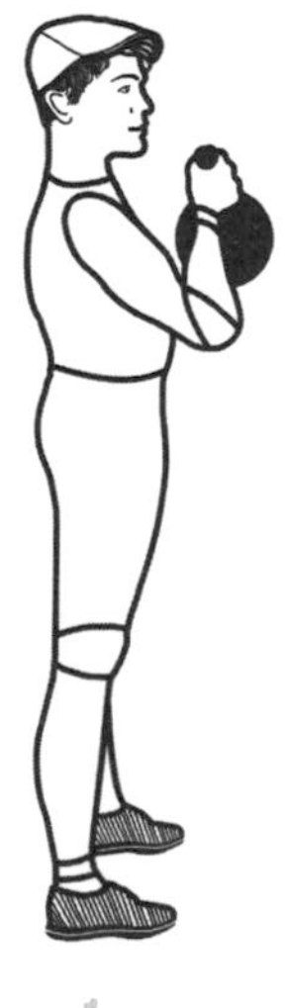

1

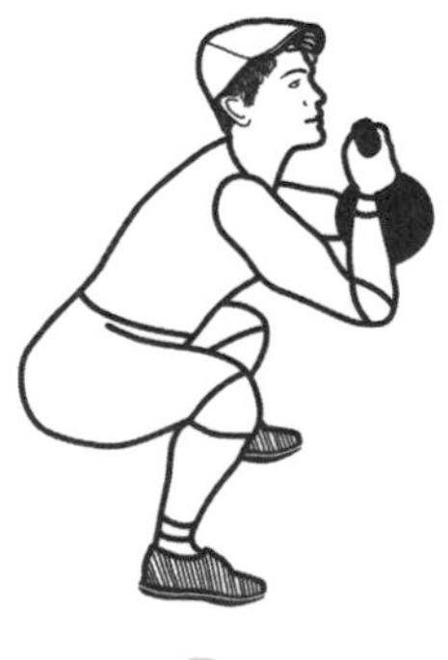

2

66 Kettlebell snatch

A snatch combines a one-hand swing with a momentum-assisted flip—actually flipping the kettlebell over so that the handle is up and the round bell is down. The tricky part is transitioning from the top of the swing to the flip. Practice the form with your lightest kettlebell. During this and all kettlebell exercises, keep your fist in line with your forearm; and when you snatch, remove your watch or wear the face inside your wrist so you don't smash it.

Grab the kettlebell with the handle forward, and with one hand, swing it to shoulder height a few times to warm up and get in the groove. 1

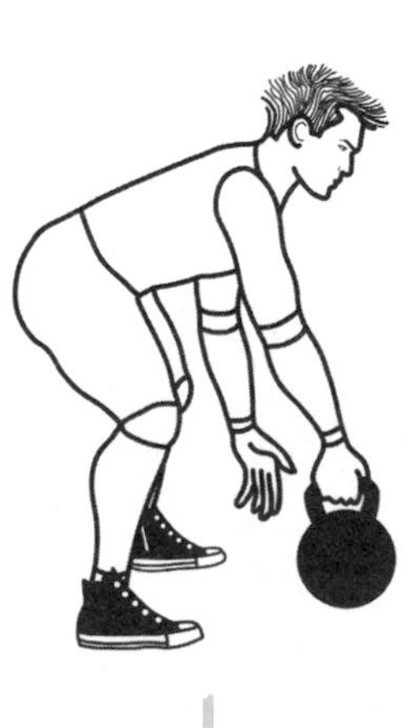

1

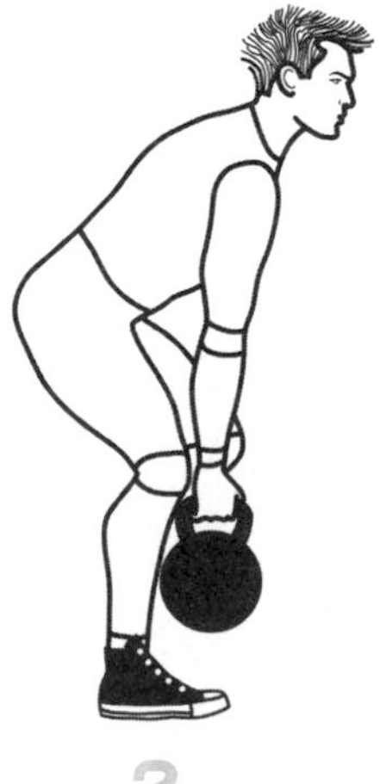

2

Now put more oomph into your legs and hips, thrust to generate more speed, and continue the swing to eye height. Do about 10 more of these with each arm. Now you're ready to snatch. 2 3

Swing the kettlebell, and as it reaches shoulder height, rotate your shoulder back and pull it in slightly to change its trajectory. A little coercion is enough. Your arm should stay nearly straight. 4

Now it gets tricky. (CONTINUED NEXT PAGE)

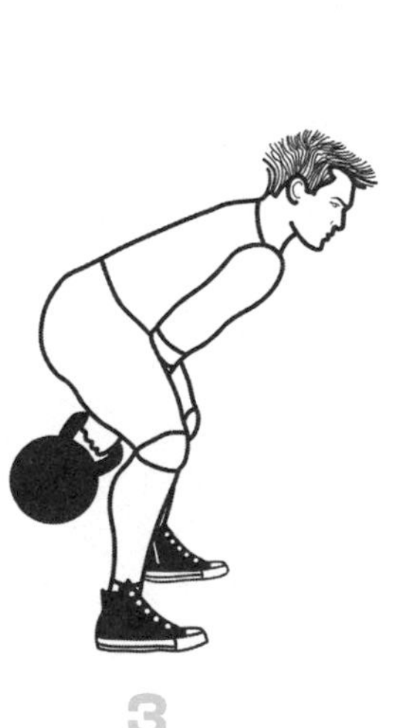

3

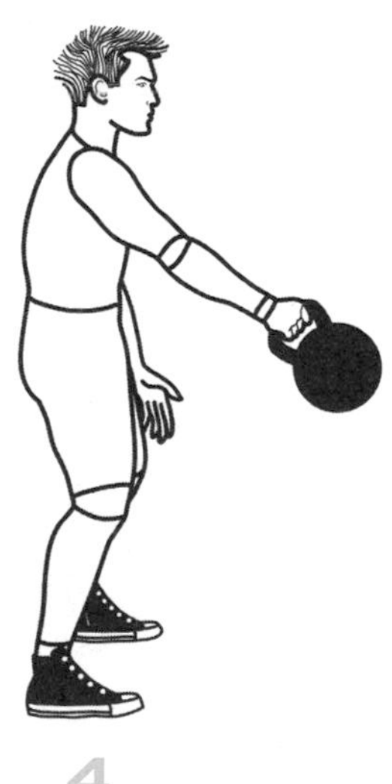

4

You've pulled it a bit closer with a subtle shoulder pull, and as it swings above your shoulder, smoothly push your hand through the handle and pull it inward a bit more. Then transition to a momentum-assisted swing-plus-press to straighten your arm and lock it in place while it's over your head. Done right, the kettlebell won't pound your wrist. 5 6

Then let it drop down in a swing, and do another. One arm at a time, start light to learn good form, then add weight and work up to sets of 10. If you can do more than that, you can snatch a heavier weight.

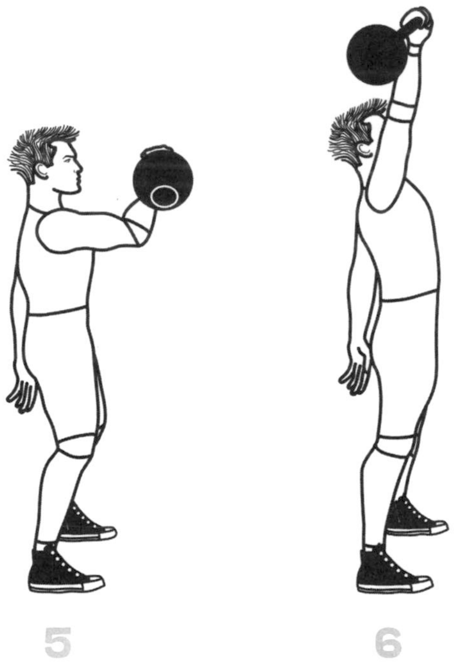

67 Kettlebell Turkish get-up

This classic kettlebell exercise gives you invincible shoulders, and is the most awkward way to lift weight ever invented. The threat of injury from dropping the kettlebell is ever present, so don't try this until you're comfortable and confident with the other kettlebell exercises.

Start with a 5- or 10-pound bell, until your form and strength can handle more. Don't push your weight limits with get-ups; always stay in control.

- Lie on your back, kettlebell on your right side, outside your shoulder. 1
- Roll to the right, grab the kettlebell with both hands, and roll back with it, resting it above your shoulder, and with your left arm straight, out to the side, palm down. 2 3
- Keep your left leg straight, and bend your right knee about 90 degrees, foot on the floor. Press the kettlebell straight up with your right arm. 4
- Roll left, using your left arm as a brace and triangulating into a half-sit. All this time, the right arm is straight up, holding the kettlebell. You're about to get halfway up.
- Shift your body slightly forward while you bend and swing your left leg rearward, your left foot swinging past your right heel, finishing this step sitting more upright, balanced on your left knee. All this time your right arm still holds that kettlebell straight up. 5

- Using your left knee as support, like a pontoon, push up with your right leg until you're standing, still holding the kettlebell straight up, like a Turk. 6 7

To reverse it:

- Go down onto your left knee.
- Brace yourself with your left arm while you:
    * Swing your left foot forward to its starting position.
    * Lower your torso so you're lying on your back in the starting position. That's one complete get-up.

Keeping the weight straight up is key. If the weight leans, it can fall and can hurt you. I repeat, do this with a very light weight until you know exactly what you're doing, then gradually work up to heavier ones.

Work up to 5 in a row per side. Eventually, if you can do 20 percent of your body weight, that's great; 25 percent is really impressive; 30 percent is getting into Russian territory.

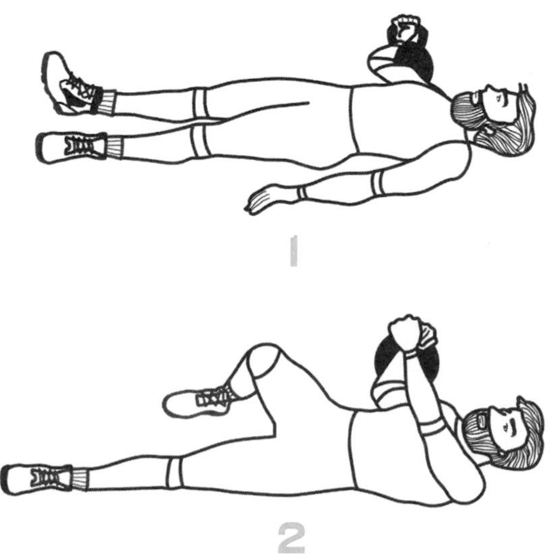

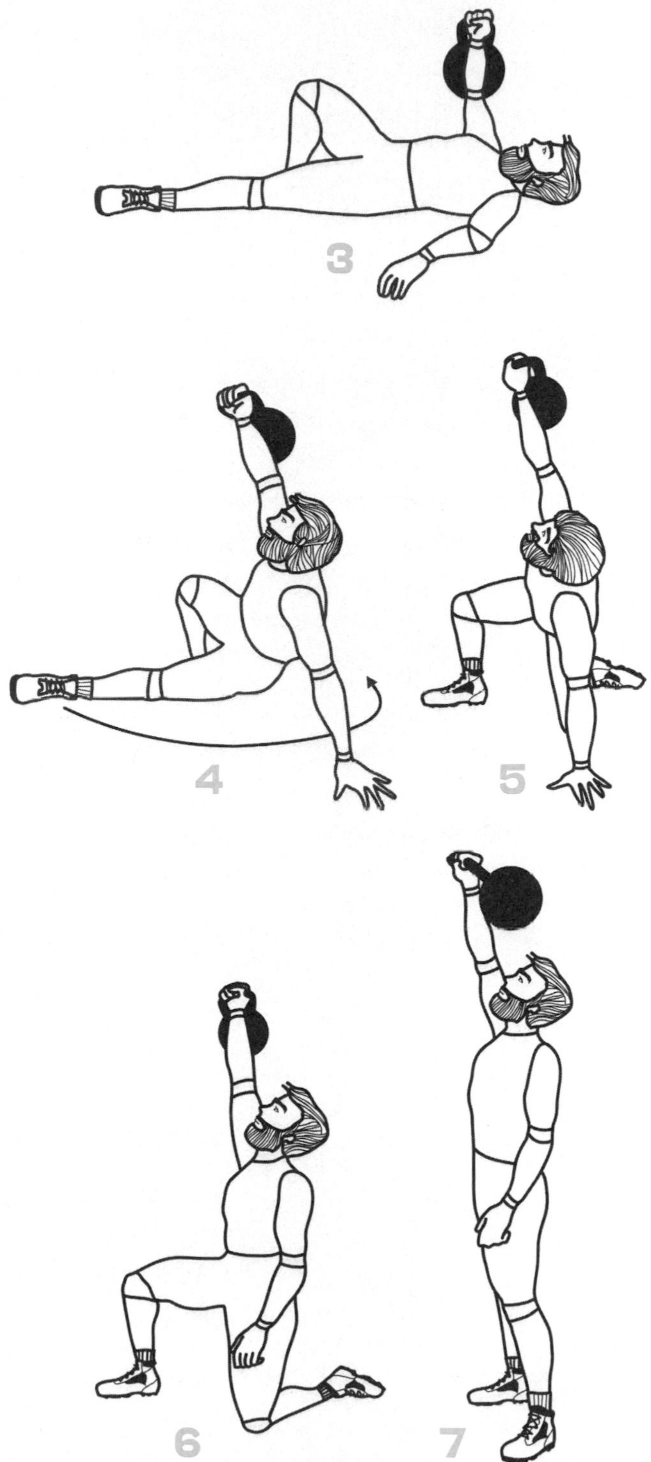
3
4
5
6
7

68 Kettlebell clean, squat, press

This may be the best kettlebell exercise of all, because it's three exercises in one.

You know what a squat and press are. "Clean" is a weight lifter's term for moving a weight from the floor to the waist, then up to the chest, with your hands in front of your shoulders, palms up. The movement has the same ending position as a weight-lifting clean, but in this exercise, you swing it up there, instead of lifting it. The illustrations show two kettlebells, but start out with one and move up to two when you're ready.

THE CLEAN:

Start with a wider-than-shoulders stance, the kettlebell about 6 inches in front of your feet. 1

Pick up the kettlebell with two hands and let it swing back automatically, as with a two-hand swing. 2

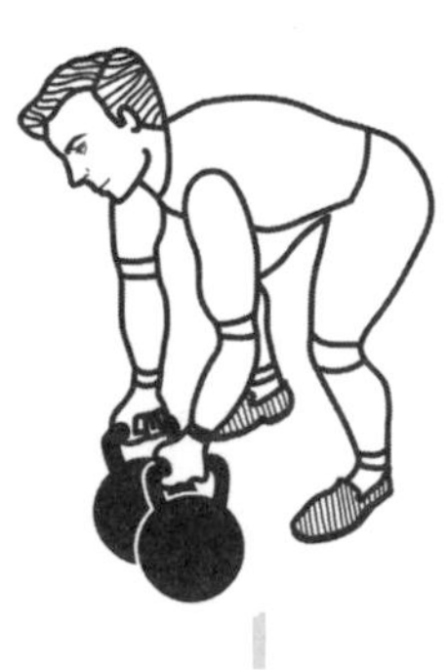

1

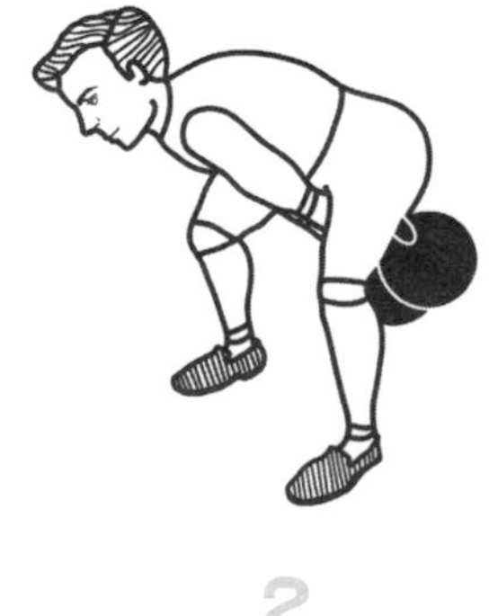

2

Once it's behind you, use your legs and hip thrusts to lift it to about shoulder height. 3

As it nears the top, pull it in, catch it in front of your chest while flexing your knees as though you're catching a water balloon or a blob of jelly. 4 5 Your wrist should be in line with your forearm, your hands in front of your chest toward the center, with the kettlebell resting on the back of your lower arm.

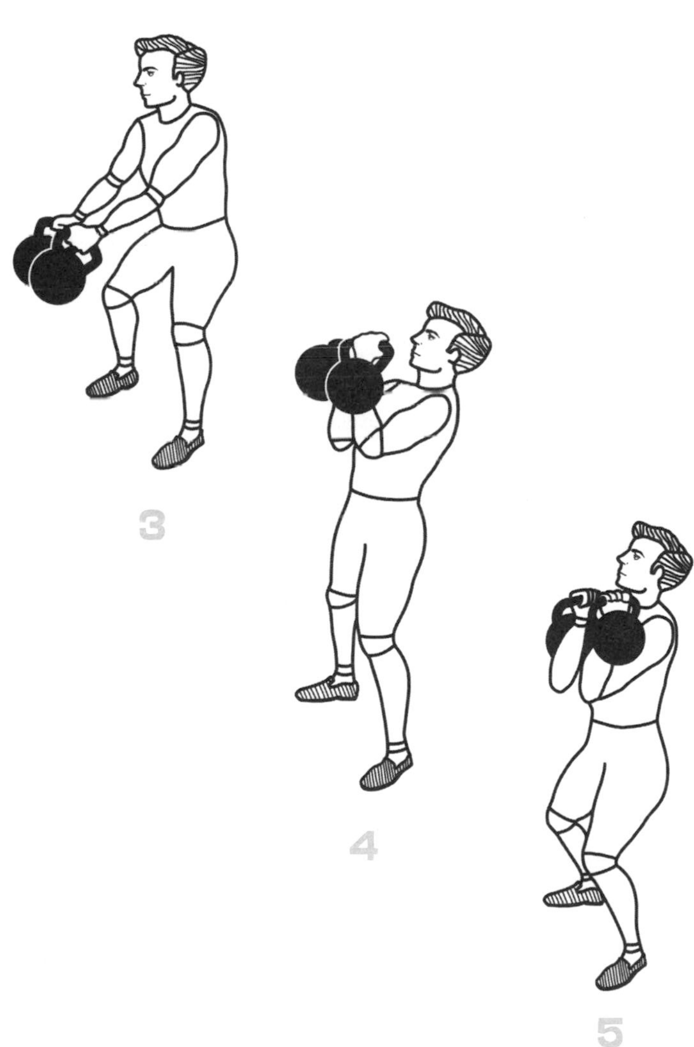

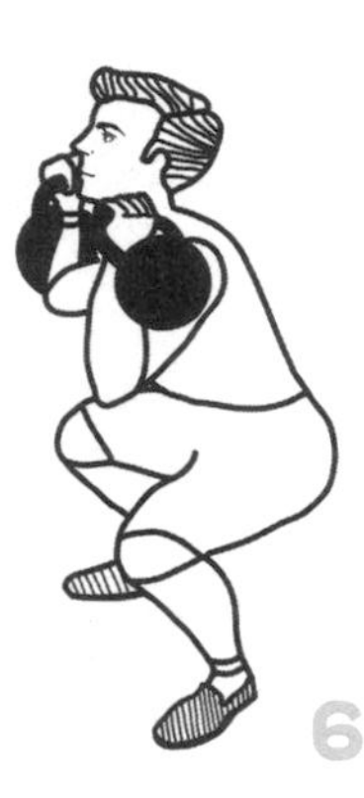

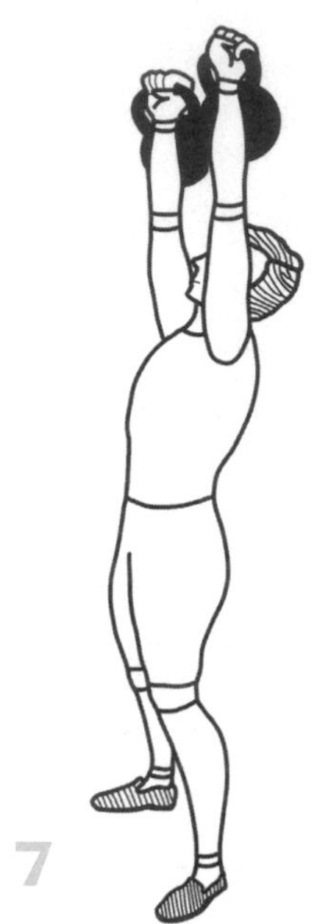

THE SQUAT:

Now just dip into a proper squat—butt back, weight on the back of your feet, shins nearly vertical. 6

THE PRESS:

As you rise from the squat, press the bell upward just before your legs are straight. The momentum generated by your legs helps push it to the top. 7

Then let it fall in a controlled drop, completing it with a rearward swing between your legs, which leads you into the next swing-to-clean. 8 9 10

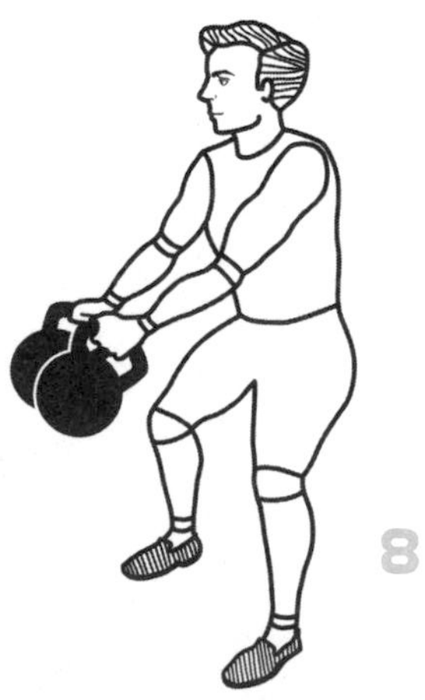

When you've perfected the move with one kettlebell, try two bells of the same weight at the same time. Do sets of 5 to 15, depending on the weight. If you rest a few minutes after the first set, the second set will be easier because your muscles will be warmed up and ready for more action.

VARIATIONS:

- Forget the clean; just squat and press.
- Forget the squat; just clean and press.
- Use a lighter weight, and for the squat and press, slow down to half your speed.

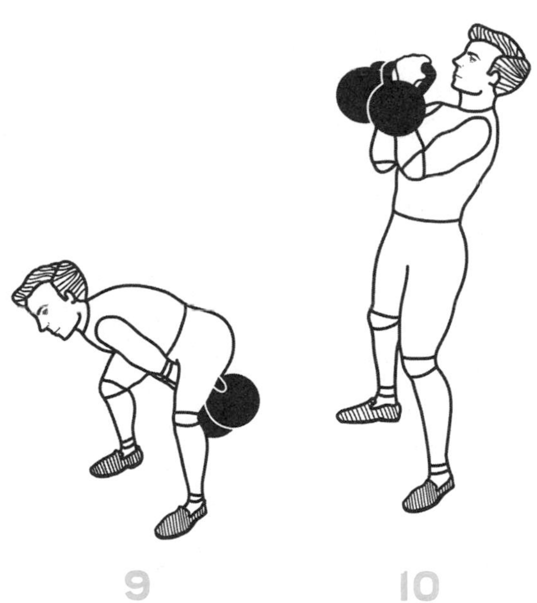

9 10

69 Windmills, with and without a kettlebell

The windmill strengthens your core and prevents lower back injuries, and will keep your back strong and pain-free as you age. If it's too late for that, stick with two-hand swings until your back feels good, and then tackle the windmill. Learn it with no weight, and when you're ready for weights, start with 5- to 10-pounders.

WINDMILLS WITHOUT WEIGHT

Stand with your feet about 4 inches wider than your shoulders, toes pointed a bit outward.

With your left hand aimed at the ceiling and your right arm hanging down naturally, shift your toes a bit to the right, bend to the right, and steer your right hand just inside your right knee. It's OK to bend your right knee a bit extra as you go down.

Look up as you go down and try to touch the floor with your fingertips. Looking up helps keep your high arm vertical, the only way it can support weight later on when you add a kettlebell.

Once you're as low as you can go, stand upright while curling your right hand upward (point it toward the ceiling), while shifting your toes to the left and bringing your left hand down, arm inside that bent knee again. When you're as low as you can get, reverse to an upright, keeping your arms in a windmill position.

Work up to 10 per side alternating left and right, and do them at least once a month, twice at most.

WINDMILLS WITH ONE KETTLEBELL

Grip your kettlebell with your right hand and stand up straight, feet about 4 inches wider than your shoulders. 1

As you lower your kettlebell toward the inside of your right foot, raise your left hand and follow it with your eyes. 2

Once you're as low as you can go, come back up again by bending your elbow and curling the kettlebell up as you start to lower the opposite arm. 3

As you straighten up, raise the kettlebell slowly up over your head and lower your opposite hand toward the ground inside your knee and foot. 4

Continue down to as low as you can go with your free hand. 5

Switch arms after each complete cycle.

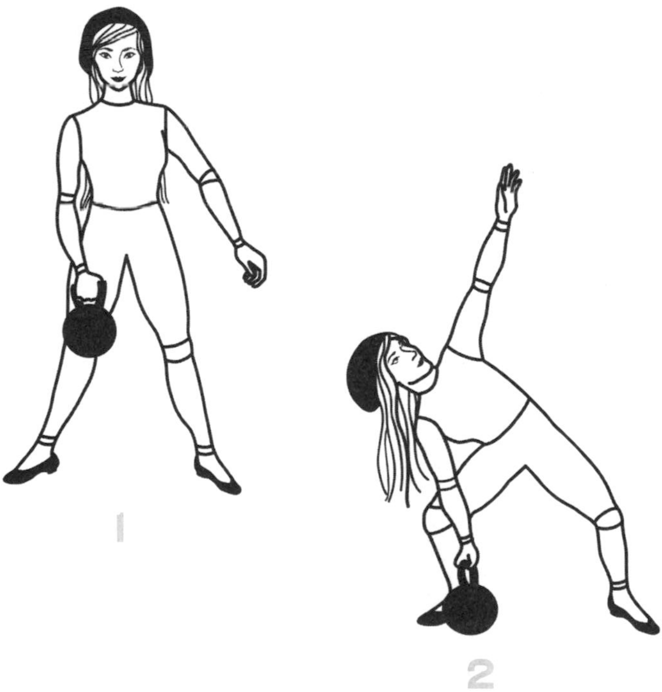

WINDMILLS WITH TWO KETTLEBELLS

The form is exactly the same, and it's not much harder, because the kettlebells hang lower than your fingers can reach, so they hit the floor before your fingertips would, which means less awkward leaning for you. When the kettlebell is touching the floor and your next move is to straighten up, curl the lower kettlebell as you straighten and as your left hand descends. They pass by each other on opposite sides of the body, one passing inside your knee while you press the other upward.

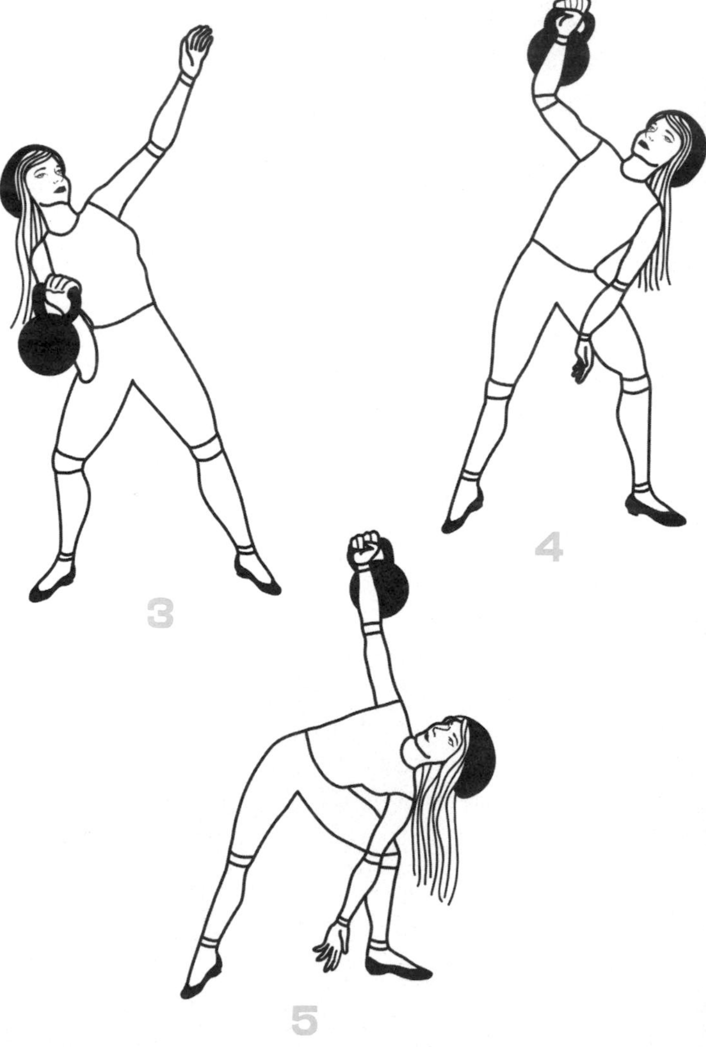

70 The brutal Tabata

Izumi Tabata was a Japanese Olympic speed-skating coach in 1996 when he was credited with developing a high-intensity, 4-minute workout that provides all the aerobic benefit of a 45-minute, huffy-puffy training effort in less than one-tenth of the time, and with less risk for injury. A Tabata is eight 20-second all-out efforts separated by 10 seconds of rest. Like this:

20 seconds all out / 10 seconds rest

20 seconds all out / 10 seconds rest

20 seconds all out / 10 seconds rest

20 seconds all out / 10 seconds rest

20 seconds all out / 10 seconds rest

20 seconds all out / 10 seconds rest

20 seconds all out / 10 seconds rest

20 seconds all out / 10 seconds rest

This Tabata adds up to (20 seconds all out + 10 seconds rest) × 8.

Although the all-out time is only 160 seconds, it's a tough 160 seconds, since the rest periods aren't enough for you to even begin to catch your breath. That's why it works, and why it's so brutal.

You can do Tabata running sprints, burpees, standing long jumps, rowing, sprinting up hills on a bike, pedaling a stationary bike, or any combination of exercises that gets the muscles burning and your lungs gasping for more oxygen. You can do all one exercise or mix it up. The point is to burn and gasp for 2 minutes and 40 seconds.

A full Tabata, as described, will be too hard unless you're already fit and used to burning and gasping, so start with 10 seconds on, 30 seconds off and 6 reps. Every two weeks, increase your "on" time and shorten your rest time until you're at 20 seconds and 10 seconds. Then work on your reps. Don't give up on Tabatas just because you can't do 8 reps of 20 on, 10 off on your first try. Dilute it at first, and work toward a full one.

I find this interesting: According to Izumi Tabata himself, the full workout named for him was actually developed by the speed-skating team's head coach, Irisawa Koichi. How it came to be called Tabata is inaccessible history for now—maybe it was the first reporter's flub—but it's nice that Tabata credits Koichi.

71 Killer burpees

Burpees—also called squat-thrusts—are the most exhausting all-around workout you can get with body weight alone. They use more muscles than any other exercise, and they mix stretching and explosive compressions, extensions, and jumps. They'll get you gassed real fast. If you can do burpees, you can do anything. Here's how:

- Stand with your feet about shoulder-width apart. 1
- Squat, hands on the ground, usually outside your knees. 2

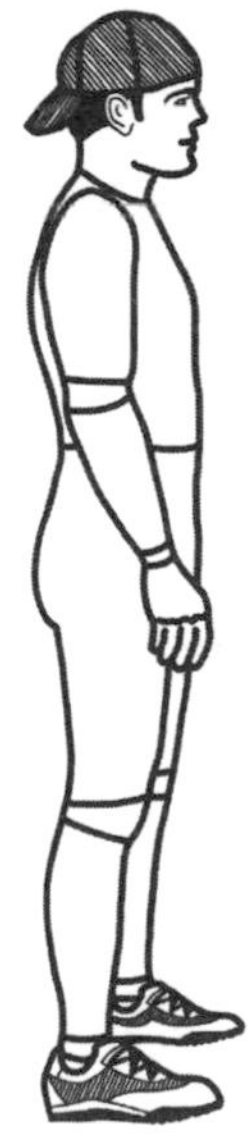

1

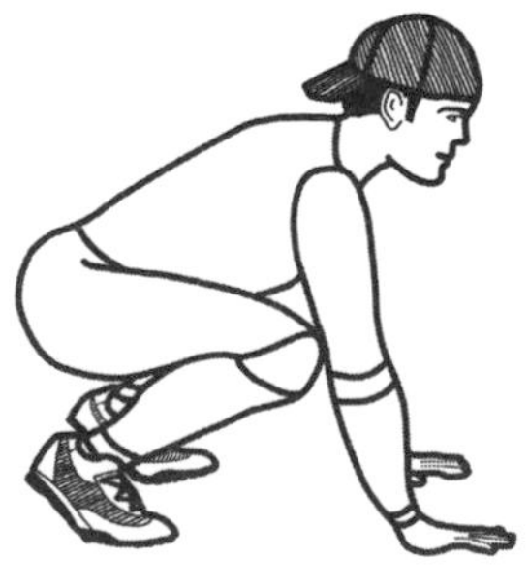

2

- Kick your feet rearward and catch yourself in a push-up's UP position. 3
- Lower yourself to the push-up's DOWN position. 4
- Then push yourself back up (you've just done a push-up). 5
- Reverse-thrust your feet forward to a squat.
- Jump up so your feet clear the ground. 6

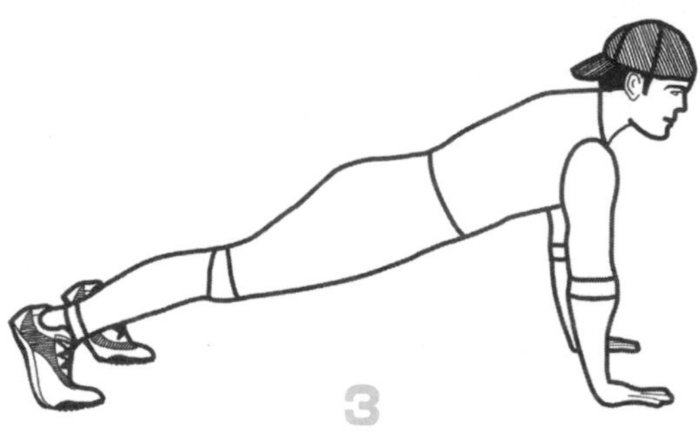

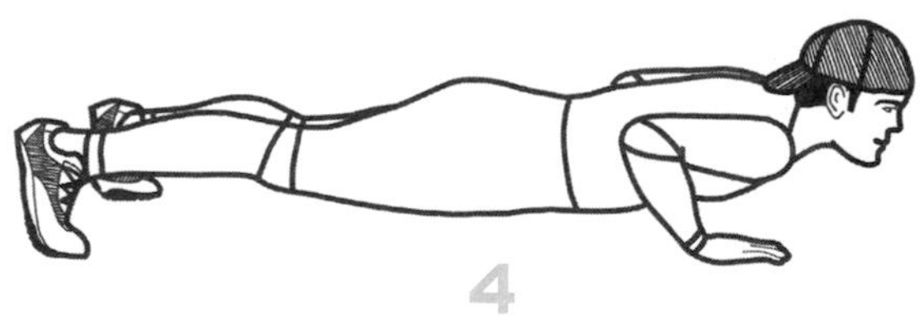

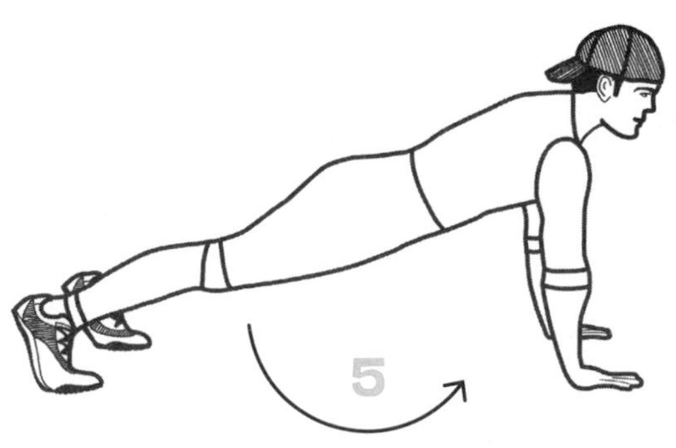

This is a 6-count burpee; a 4-counter eliminates the push-up (steps 3 and 4). If you can't do push-ups, do 4-count burpees until you can. A small minority consider a burpee proper only when you raise your hands over your head on the jump, but I'm not among them. When you do enough burpees, you will achieve the only goal that matters: a workout so complete you're done in minutes, gasping for air and so tired you can barely stand up.

Burpees, the two-hand kettlebell swing, and the kettlebell clean, squat, press are the most all-around beneficial exercises in this book. Combine them into your own 3-minute routine, and you'll rule the world in a few months.

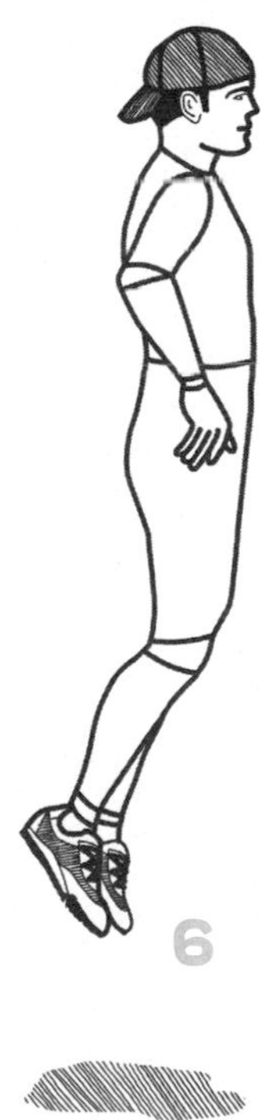

72 Countdowns

Start with 6 to 10 reps of any grunty exercise (squats, push-ups, kettlebell anything) or an explosive, gaspy one (burpees, kangaroos). After the first set, rest 10 to 30 seconds, then do one less of the same thing, and repeat down to zero. Rest only enough in order to complete the next set, whether it's 10 seconds or a minute. Each set should be about as hard as the one before it.

Countdowns give one set of muscles a killer workout, but you can mix up the exercises here, too. To vary it, you can count down by odd numbers or evens. The goal is the same as always: burning muscles, gasping breath, hating the moment, but getting through it quickly.

The hardest countdowns for me are burpees with a kangaroo thrown in on the jump-up. Any countdown involving burpees is supertough—and beneficial. Here are two options:

ONE OPTION:

10 burpees / rest
9 burpees / rest
8 burpees / rest
7 burpees / rest
6 burpees / rest
5 burpees / rest
4 burpees / rest
3 burpees / rest
2 burpees / rest
1 burpee

ANOTHER OPTION:

10 squats (with or without weight) / rest
9 squats / rest
8 squats / rest
7 push-ups / rest
6 squats / rest
5 push-ups / rest
4 squats / rest
3 push-ups / rest
2 squats / rest
1 push-up

73 Repetitive countdowns

Pick four exercises—burpees, push-ups, sit-ups, kettlebell snatches—any combination that engages most or all of your muscles. Do them as fast as you can—first a set of 8 reps of each, then a set of 6, then a set of 4. That's 72 reps, a full day's workout. Rest minimally between sets—about 10 seconds. Rest a few seconds more if you need to, but don't catch your breath. Keep it hard.

VARIATIONS:

10 reps + 8 reps + 6 reps x 4 different exercises = 96 reps

9 reps + 7 reps + 5 reps x 3 different exercises = 63 reps

The goal is to move for 3 to 7 minutes, breathing hard and straining muscles the whole time. Try to maintain decent form, but allow yourself to get a little sloppy as your muscles fatigue. This breaks the "go slow" rule, but here you're after a high heart-rate workout rather than pure strength building.

OTHER POSSIBILITIES:

8 burpees + 8 squats + 8 kangaroos + 8 push-ups

6 burpees + 6 squats + 6 kangaroos + 6 push-ups

4 burpees + 4 squats + 4 kangaroos + 4 push-ups

In these or any speed exercises, I like to do body weight–only exercises, because there's less risk of injury if your form goes to hell when you're fatigued.

74 Fibonacci

Here's another workout-by-the-numbers.

Fibonacci numbers are a sequence created by adding the last two consecutive numbers to get the next one, like this: 0, 1, 1, 2, 3, 5, 8, 13, 21, 34, 55, 89, 144.

In the Fibonacci sequence, any two consecutive numbers add up to the next one. There's no magic or voodoo factor to Fibonacci numbers. They're just another way to pull you through a workout. Here are some sequences that work for my friends and me:

FIBONACCI PYRAMIDS (AKA FIBOMIDS)

You start low, climb up, and descend again, resting minimally between sets.

3 push-ups

5 push-ups

8 kangaroos

13 squats

21 squats

13 push-ups

8 kangaroos

5 burpees

That's 76 reps. Fill in your own exercise, or do all of the same one. No matter what you do, it'll be hard enough.

You can reverse the pattern to do Fibovalleys—starting high, working down, and then working back up, like this: 21-13-8-5-8-13-21. That's 89 reps.

This sequence is ideal for two-hand kettlebell swings, an all-body exercise.

WHO WAS FIBONACCI AND WHAT'S SO SPECIAL ABOUT HIS NUMBERS?

Fibonacci was an Italian mathematician who lived from 1170 to about 1250. He was also known as Leonardo Pisano and Leonardo of Pisa.

Fibonacci numbers and the proportions derived from them are found in shell and flower patterns, ferns, Greek architecture, and the human body. The ratio of one fibo-number to the next in the sequence is roughly 1 to 1.618. Rectangles with these proportions are known as golden rectangles. When you remove a square from one, the remaining rectangle is also golden—1 to 1.618. Connecting the intersections of the lines forms a Golden Spiral, which grows in the same 1 to 1.618 proportions with every 90° turn.

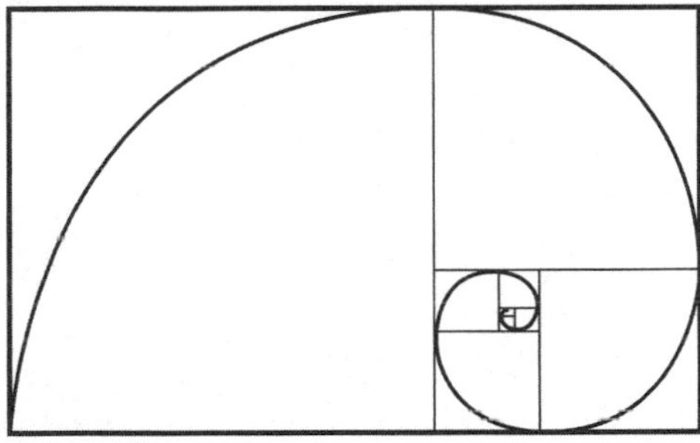

From fingertip to wrist, the bones grow in Golden Ratio proportions. The ratio of hand length (tip of middle finger to wrist) to forearm length (wrist to elbow) is also Golden.

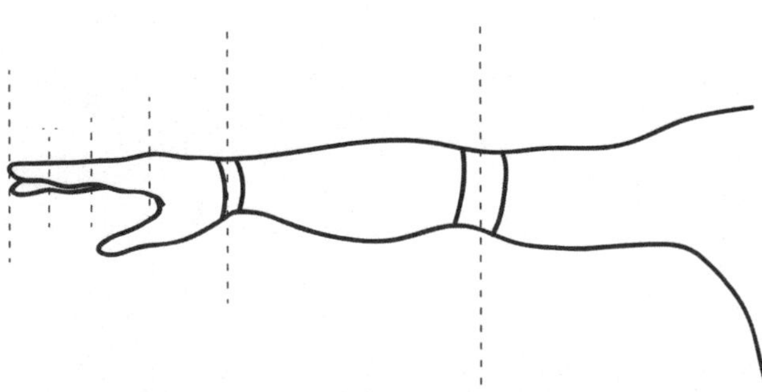

75 Using the potentially deadly ab wheel

An ab wheel is one of those wheels with handles that you see on late-night infomercials, in some gyms, and in many fitness equipment stores. Ab stands for abdominal. If you use it incorrectly, it can give you a hernia and wreck your lower back, but when you use it the right way, it'll harden your stomach, protect you from hernias, and strengthen your lower back. Don't go near an ab wheel if you already have a hernia or a damaged lower back.

Kneel with a wall about 3 feet in front of you, and slowly roll into it. Concentrate on arching your back outward, like a dolphin's back, to reduce lower back stress. 1 Then roll backward to the start position. Repeat up to 15 times. That's plenty.

Once you're rolling nearly full length (arms outstretched, little bend at the waist), do it standing up. Start with your toes about 3 feet from the wall. 2 Roll toward the wall and back, 5 to 10 times. 3 As this becomes easy, add a few inches at a time until your feet are almost as far from the wall as you are tall. Show-offs on YouTube extend out fully, but that's a risky party trick.

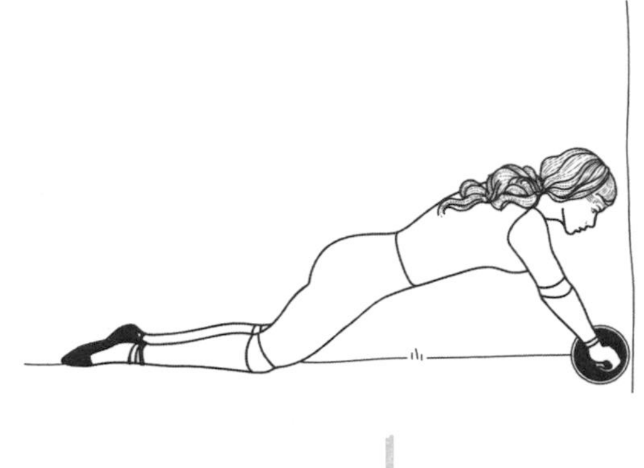

1

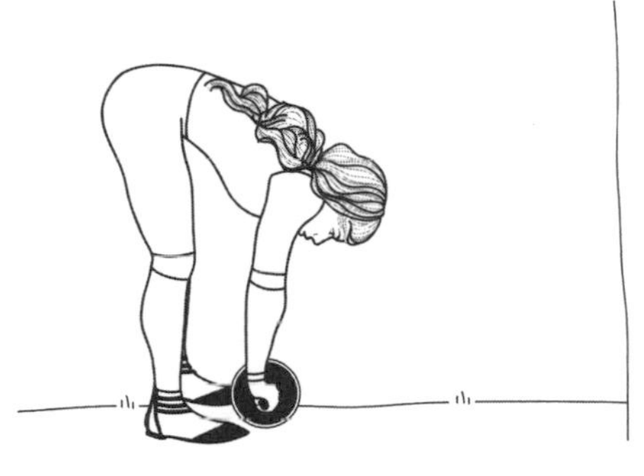

2

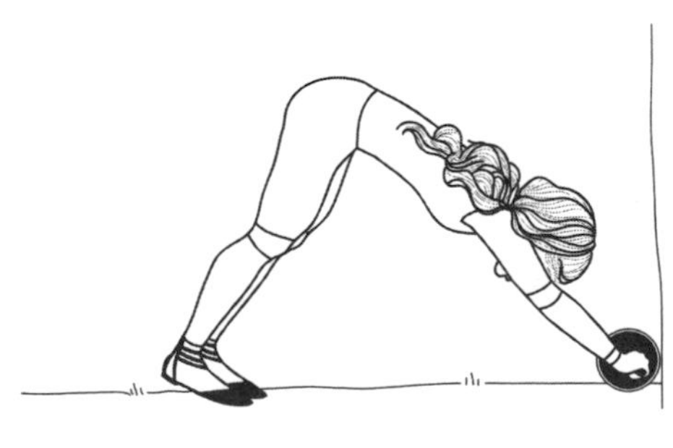

3

76 Medicine ball fetch

Medicine balls have been used as training devices since the Greeks invented them almost 2,000 years ago, and now you can buy them anywhere exercise gear is sold. The most common medicine ball workout is "wall ball," where you toss it high against a wall, catch it as you go into a squat, then spring up and repeat. That's a good one, but I like fetch better, which is to say, I hate it more while doing it, but it helps more muscles and gets me gasping harder than wall ball does.

You'll need one or two medicine balls—about $20 to $45 each. If you're just starting out, get 4- to 8-pounders, and if you're strong, 10- to 15-pounders.

Go to a football field with a track around it. First, see how fast you can cover 100 yards on the field by throwing and chasing, throwing and chasing from goal line to goal line. Throw underhand, overhand, backward over your head, forward over your head, one hand or two, and one ball or two. It's a freestyle exercise. The first few times you do it, mix up your throws to vary the muscles you're working. Do this a few times over a period of a week or two, and if your lower back is fine the morning after, take it to the track outside the field and see how far you can go in 4 minutes. Or see how long it takes to play fetch for a whole 400 meters.

This is a great aerobic/anaerobic/all-muscle option for a full-day's workout in a few minutes, with great results. Four minutes of this and you're done for the day. Anything else is gravy, but don't feel like you need to do more.

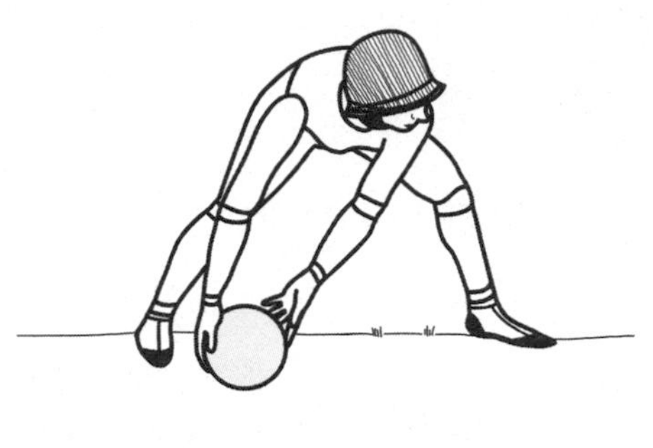

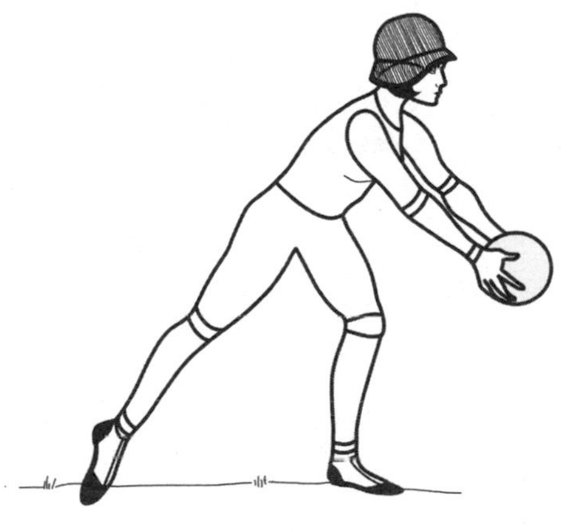

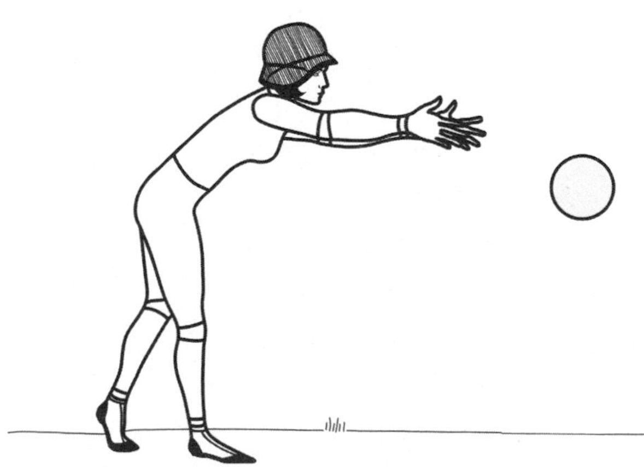

77 Sprint without pulling up lame

Sprinting is an all-out, extreme range-of-motion exercise that often punishes imperfect form, and unless you're a thief or on a team in a league, maybe you haven't sprinted since you played your last game of tag. Law-abiding adults who don't play on a team or compete on the track can go forever without sprinting.

If you just dive into sprinting, you'll pull something and disable yourself for weeks. Sprint only after you've been consistently working out for a few months and some of what you've been doing involves running—like medicine ball fetch, burpee sprints (different from the kind of sprints I'm talking about now), uphill runs alongside your bicycle, and now and then chasing a football or a Frisbee. Even then, you'll still need to warm up more than is necessary for any other exercise in this book or you'll pull a muscle. Here's a good way to warm up for a sprint:

- Walk for 5 minutes, mixing in about 30 lunges (long step with right leg, pause and almost touch the ground with your left knee, keeping your right shin as vertical as you can, then repeat, making sure you do about 15 right-foot steps and then 15 left-foot steps).
- Jog 3 minutes, some of it backward, to stretch your calves and Achilles tendons.
- Run in place with high knees and exaggerated arm movements (bring your hands from hip height to ear height) to balance the exaggerated leg movements. You want your muscles and joints to be used to a greater range of motion before you sprint.

- Run sideways, lifting your knees high and crossing your legs at each step. Again, focus not on speed but on range of movement. This limbers you up and readies your joints for the shock of the sprint.
- Do about 5 half-speed runs of 40 yards or so, resting or walking 30 seconds between efforts. This gets you used to the general motion at a safe speed.
- Then do 5 more runs at three-quarter speed. This ramps it up before the final effort.

All of this should take you about 15 minutes and feel like a workout in itself. Then you're ready to sprint.

You can sprint on a track, a football field, or between telephone poles and manhole covers on the neighborhood streets, if traffic allows. Sprint from the door handle on the Karmann Ghia to the bumper on the Subaru, then walk to the taillights on the Prelude and sprint to the trunk of the big tree. If you're on a football field, start with 40-yard sprints. If you're on the street, estimate the distance. You're aiming for a 7- to 11-second sprint at full throttle.

After your first sprint, walk for a minute or two or three, and repeat. Once your total all-out sprint time is 1½ minutes, you're done for the day. It's a hellish minute and a half, but the worst part is the warm-up. You may be sore for a few days, but it'll go away, and if you sprint once a week you'll be sore-proof.

The longest time you'll ever want to sprint during contrived exercise is about half a minute. You can't maintain good form and an all-out effort much longer than that. On a standard 400-meter track, see how long it takes you to run 100 meters, 150 meters, or 200 meters. But start shorter to get your form and sprint-fitness down.

78 Any hill in your neighborhood is like a free public gym

The difference in effort between moving on flat ground and moving up a hill is tremendous. You can see that when you roll a ball or ride a bike, so take advantage of it.

Running up hills gets a separate entry from flat-ground sprints, because it feels so different. They both help your heart and muscles way more than a 2-hour jog; they don't punish you for bad form as much as flat-track sprints do, because your leg speed is so much slower, so you're less likely to trip or pull something. There's more risk of straining a calf muscle, though, so prepare for hill sprints by walking up the hill a few times first, walking down it backward, and then maybe jogging up it for 10 to 20 seconds at a time. When you're stretched and warm, you're ready.

Find a gradual hill that takes about 15 to 20 seconds to run up at full speed. Walk down (backward for part of it to stretch those calves), then repeat 6 to 8 times, or until you've sprinted at least 2½ minutes and at most 4—that's more than plenty. Go to steeper hills only after you've had a few rounds over a few weeks with the easier hills, to make sure your calves are ready for the extra strain that comes with steepness.

79 Turning your bicycle into exercise gear

Bicycles and bike riding are my main thing, and the fun skyrocketed when I quit relying on my bike for exercise. Riding *is* exercise, but when you rely on it for fitness, you lose out on the fun of riding a bike, and you don't get an all-over workout—just look at the arms of pro cyclists. But you can work out on your bike if you give up the idea of having a fun time while you're doing it. One of the benefits to this way of thinking is that you'll appreciate your normal rides so much more.

HERE ARE TWO WAYS TO USE YOUR BIKE FOR A REAL WORKOUT:

- Hill intervals: If you live in hilly country, pick out a fine one that would take you 20 seconds to 1 minute to climb, and climb it repeatedly, 5 to 8 times, as hard as you can.
- On-and-offs: On a ride with several short climbs, hop off your bike and run up some of them, pushing your bike alongside as you go. On short, steep hills, you can probably run up them while pushing your bike faster than you can pedal up them. It keeps your running muscles in decent form and activates more muscles than just riding does.

80 Hotel exercising

- Use the pool. I like to swim, but my work and life haven't allowed me to cross over the line yet to become "a swimmer," so I just swim when I travel. Many hotels that aren't in New York City have pools, and they're usually empty in the mornings. Swimming violates the "if it's not dreadful, it's not efficient" rule, but it's a good break from the intense, burning, gasping routines I usually recommend. It's all-body, a great way to recuperate and relax, and it feels natural. I'm not changing my tune. If you let swimming dominate your exercise time, and continue to eat carbs, you'll spend a hell of a lot of time in the water without a lot to show for it. But as an exercise to do every now and then, it's great.
- Take the stairs. Climbing stairs is like doing continuous fast, one-legged squats, especially if you skip every other step. Set a goal—20 flights, for instance. Climb 5 to 10 flights of stairs, take the elevator back down, and repeat until you've reached your goal. If 20 is easy, do 40, 60, 80, or more. Check into tall hotels.
- You can also climb stairs slowly. Stepping on every other step, push up as slowly as you can, while maintaining balance. Get the burn going and maintain it as long as you can, up to 5 or 6 minutes. You could just do slow squats in your room, but giving yourself distance to cover and floors to climb is mentally easier and physically just as good.

81 On tired or lazy days, spread it out

Some days it's emotionally just too hard to do even 3 consecutive intense minutes of anything. You've got stuff on your mind, you're too busy, you're sore, whatever—the intensity is like kicking yourself when you're down, but you still want to do something, so do this:

Pick a number between 50 and 75 and do that many reps of a variety of exercises, and give yourself all day to do it. Do 5 to 20 sets of any exercise in this book, or any other you feel like. Do 5 push-ups at 9 a.m., 10 burpees at noon, 15 squats at 12:30, 10 more burpees at 2 p.m., 20 kettlebell two-hand swings at 4 p.m., and 5 burpees after dinner. That's 65 reps, and it was easy—nothing took more than 1 minute, most took way less, and you got to rest immediately after. Have easy days like this once or twice a week. If you're coming off a sedentary life, you might want to work out this way up to four times a week. Once you're stronger and fitter, it's fine to alternate days like this with compact 3-to-7-minute no-rest exercise bursts.

WHAT'S GOING ON INSIDE?

If you're like most people, you know more inconsequential facts about celebrities than useful facts about your insides. That's potentially tragic, but by reading this chapter, you're taking the first step to having at least a balance of the two. In it, you'll find descriptions of some pre-historical events that I didn't witness and processes inside our bodies that I've never seen. But the great thing about science is that when the facts have been revealed, they are no less true whether bellowed by a scientist, scribbled by a medical professional, or muttered by a lunatic. I'm somewhere in the middle, and I think you'll come out of this chapter with fun facts about guts, and an understanding that will inspire you to cut back on the carbs.

82 Ape + fish and fat + 2.8 million years = you

About 3 million years ago, climate change led to a loss of jungle habitat and forced apes into the African woodlands, where they had to find new food to eat. Right off the bat, they also discovered they *were* food for the many large, fast, toothy carnivores. The displaced ape ate roots and shoots near the water and, over time, added raw meat stolen from lion kills, and, most important, fish and shellfish. It was food an ape could gather with lower risk; that even a young ape could pluck out of the water. As his head and guts were adapting to the softer, more digestible food, he lost gut yardage no longer needed to digest plant roughage, and over time, his rib cage shrank accordingly. His earlier massive jaw muscles shrank because the extra strength was no longer necessary, and his attachment point to the head lowered, compressing his skull less with each chew. This allowed the skull to expand, making room for a bigger brain—which grew from the fattier diet of mammals and fish rich in the right nutrients required to grow a more complex brain.

After eating this digestible, nutrient-dense diet for several hundred thousand years, the ape changed enough to be deemed a new species—*Australopithecus afarensis*, a 3½- to 4½- foot-tall humanish woodland ape that could walk on two feet (though not as well as we do) but still climbed and slept in trees like a jungle ape.

Then about 2.4 million years ago, and after about 600,000 years of survival among carnivorous predators and eating increasingly more raw meat, *Australopithecus afarensis* had evolved to become the first of our genus—*Homo*—and humans were born. The first of the new genus climbed and slept in trees like apes, but walked on two feet like we do. They were handy with crude stone tools (used to break bones, shells, and scrape off meat), so they were named *Homo habilis*, meaning handy man.

Homo habilis's food continued to be meat, most of it raw. A lot of raw mammal and shellfish meat has the consistency of tough chewing gum. It's softer than a tough root, but still requires a lot of powerful jaw action. A chimpanzee, with massive teeth and jaws, can spend 3 hours chewing 12 ounces of mammal meat, and it's just not worth the time. *Homo habilis* had smaller jaws and would have had a harder time with it, so he used tools to smash and chop and destroy the connective tissue that made it so chewy off the bone or out of the shell. Tenderizing the meat let him eat more of it with less chewing *and* increased its digestibility. Over more time, his jaw and teeth adapted to the easier food by downsizing, his rib cage lost its downward flare, and his guts shortened yet again. Adapting to life out of trees, he grew taller, his legs got longer, and his arms got shorter, so he could run upright better and live slightly less dangerously in the tall grass. That was fortuitous, because as he was evolving, he'd lost his tree-climbing skills, and was sleeping on the ground.

With tools now tenderizing the meat and a steady diet of fish and shellfish, his jaw muscles weakened more and the attachment point grew lower on the head—now approaching the top of his ears and allowing the skull to grow bigger. This, along with more and better nutrition, led to a bigger brain. Then about 1.9 million years ago, after a 500,000-year reign and eating lots of easily chewed meat, fish, and shellfish, the next *Homo* species evolved.

This species was *Homo erectus*, named because he stood like we do. Upright walking made travel easier, and though *H. erectus* evolved in Africa, some migrated out, notably north to the cold country in Europe, and others, the fossil record suggests, toward China. *Homo erectus* was the longest-surviving human of all so far—about 1.8 million years—and the first to tame fire. Fire was a big deal, since it revealed and scared away wild animals at night, *and*—more important to his continuing evolution—it cooked meat. Cooked meat is easier to chew, so *H. erectus* could eat more and digest it more easily. As a result, his body kept changing. His hips narrowed, and his intestinal mass and rib cage shrank again. And once again, the cooked, soft, high-fat food (and more fish) continued to allow jaw muscles to weaken and attach at a lower point on the head, and the skull and brain continued to grow. The bigger brain led to a more complex social life, with improved communication and more efficient group hunting. More meat

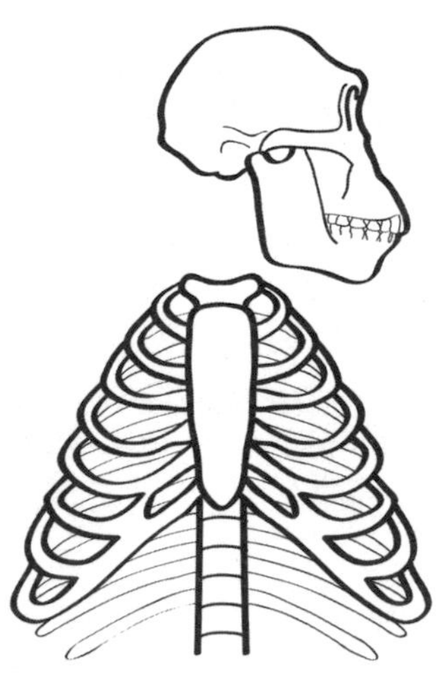

AUSTRALOPITHECUS AFARENSIS

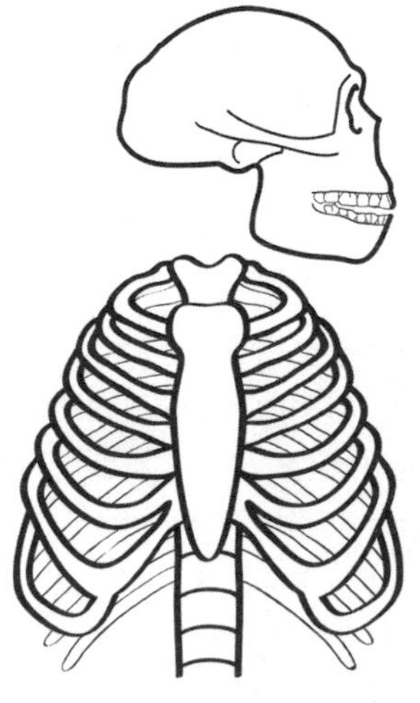

HOMO ERECTUS

in the fire led to more sophisticated cooking methods and a healthier, larger *H. erectus*. Near the end of his almost 1.8-million-year reign, the taller ones cleared 6 feet. I'm only 5 feet 9½ inches.

At this point, the evolutionary timeline gets less certain, but it's widely accepted that we—*Homo sapiens*—evolved directly from fat- and-fish-eating *Homo erectus*.

We have the small rib cages, short guts, and big heads and brains of meat eaters, and if our ancestors hadn't eaten meat and had a steady diet of the fish and shellfish that supplied the nutrients critical to brain growth, we wouldn't have become what we are. It's worth thinking about that as we debate the ethics and consequences of meat eating. If our ancestors hadn't eaten meat, we wouldn't be able to have that debate.

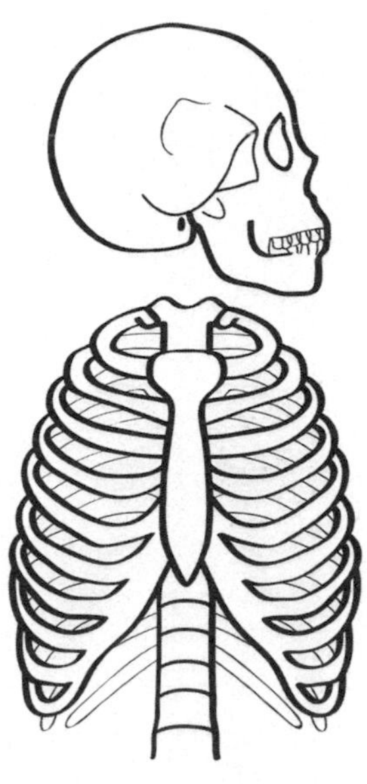

Homo sapiens

83 After millions of years of eating meat, your digestive system has grown to prefer it

Technically you're an omnivore (everything eater), which makes sense, since your ancestors were omnivorous apes. But on the way to becoming human, you ate mostly animals, and your digestive system changed from long and complex to short and simple, to better accommodate the nutrient-dense, less fibrous diet.

Meat is easy for your simple guts to digest, and the proof's in the poop; or *not*. You don't have large daily bowel movements on an all-meat diet—testimony to how thoroughly you digest meat. When your digestive system is finished with it, there's just not a lot left to make feces with. There's no indigestible fiber. There is not, as some vegetarians suggest, a dam of meat rotting in your guts—it's mush by the time it enters there. A few harmless leaves are OK—they'll be fermented in the large intestine and help feed your gut bacteria. But eat mostly meat.

84 When picking a food, go by your guts

An animal in the wild eats only the food its system has evolved to digest, because anything else kills it or makes it sick. Humans are the only animals that screw up feeding and eating. We're influenced by opinions, fads, celebrity endorsements, agendas, ethics, religion, experts, commerce, and holidays—and with all of those influences, no wonder we're confused. A lot of that could be avoided if we did like animals do and just ate the food our digestive systems evolved to process.

Here's a rundown of the four main kinds of digestive systems:

- **RUMINANT:** Animals that chew cud and have four-chambered stomachs (one of which is called the rumen) are ruminants. Deer, elephants, goats, moose, cows, and sheep are ruminants. They evolved to eat roughage, the least digestible of foods, and have a more complex digestive system to process it. Their four-chambered stomachs break down the cellulose in plants by fermenting it twice. First, it's chewed and swallowed and delivered to the rumen, a fermenting chamber that breaks it down to become cud. The cud goes to the reticulum, which drains off some liquid and sends the cud back up the esophagus for chewing. Then the rechewed cud is sent down again to the stomach. It passes through the other two chambers (omasum and abomasum), where it gets drenched in more digestive enzymes and acids before making a long trip through the small intestines, where digestion continues and nutrients are absorbed.

At the end of the small intestine, and just before the large intestine, there's a side pouch called the cecum. It's a large, second fermentation chamber to help break down the still-rough roughage. From the cecum, it makes its way to the long large intestine. At this point—after a long stay and having passed through several digesting stations and processes—the food is still only partially digested, and the considerable remainder is—in the case of cows—formed into the familiar "cow Frisbees" that dot the landscape. These results are plentiful, because ruminants have to eat constantly to even stand a chance of extracting enough nutrients from the roughage; and large, because even after all of that, digestion is still so incomplete.

- **PSEUDORUMINANT:** Pseudoruminants—among them camels, alpaca, hippos, and vicunas—aren't as good at digesting roughage as are true ruminants, because they have three, rather than four, stomach chambers; less in-stomach fermentation; and not all even chew cud. The cecum is the major fermentation site in the pseudoruminant. They need higher quality, softer roughage than the coarse fare ruminants eat.
- **AVIAN:** Avian refers to birds, but it's also the digestive system of turtles, dinosaurs, other reptiles, and some slugs. The avian mouth is toothless and bad for chewing, so an avian grabs food with its mouth and swallows it whole. The food goes undigested down the esophagus to a crop—a thin-skinned pouch that seems to herniate from the esophagus. In the crop, digestive juices soften the food, preparing it for the scrawny, twisted proventriculus—equivalent of our stomach. The proventriculus secretes enzymes to further soften the food, before sending it to the gizzard, a thick,

muscular pouch where the food is finally chewed. The gizzard is toothless, but holds intentionally swallowed rocks that combine with muscular contractions to finally chew the food. Food that's too tough or just indigestible—bones, chunks of hooves, claws, big seeds, or masses of fur and feathers—is formed into wads and gets barfed up and (if the avian is a bird) out the beak. The digestible matter passes through the small intestines and two cecums, where digestion continues, and finally passes through the large intestine and is pooped out. Since all animals with an avian digestive system eat less-fibrous, more nutrient-dense foods than do ruminants and pseudoruminants, there's no need for fermentation, cud chewing, or feces eating. The gizzard-as-mouth may not be a perfect system, but it has been sufficient for millions of years, and evolution is more about minimal requirements than perfection.

- **MONOGASTRIC:** Animals like pigs, dogs, horses, and humans have one stomach, so are "monogastric." But it is an imperfect category name, because even ruminants and pseudoruminants have just one stomach (though with several chambers). Compared to the digestive system of ruminants and pseudoruminants, the monogastric rig is much simpler, because it evolved to digest less-rough, more nutrient-dense and easily digested food.

  There are subcategories of monogastric animals, with evolutionary tweaks to their gastric systems according to their diets.

- **MONOGASTRIC CARNIVORES** (cats and dogs) chew their food only enough to mix it with saliva in order to send it down the esophagus without sticking. In the stomach, hydrochloric acid breaks down the food to mush, preparing it for more digestion and nutrient absorption in the small intestine. This is the fastest, most efficient digestion, because the food is so nutrient-dense and easily digested.

- **MONOGASTRIC HERBIVORES** (horses, guinea pigs) have longer intestines to aid the breakdown of roughage and, like ruminants and pseudoruminants, a monstrous cecum for fermenting the cellulose. On top of that, the rabbit-sized and smaller monogastric herbivores commonly eat their first passing of feces, sending it through the system a second time for further digestion.
- **HUMANS AND APES ARE MONOGASTRIC OMNIVORES** (plants or animals). But apes eat far more roughage, so have the characteristic long guts and large cecums required to digest and ferment coarse leaves and jungle foliage. Our digestive system is shorter, and what used to be a cecum has atrophied into our appendix. We don't ferment cellulose in it—it's typically about the size of a finger, too small to be a fermenting chamber, but with an opening that's easily clogged by partly digested food (and feces). That's what causes appendicitis.

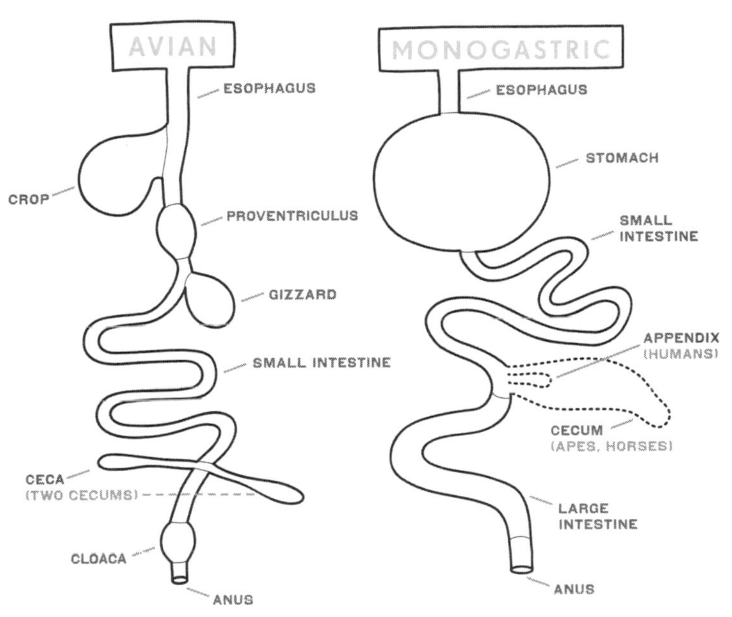
AVIAN
ESOPHAGUS
CROP
PROVENTRICULUS
GIZZARD
SMALL INTESTINE
CECA
(TWO CECUMS)
CLOACA
ANUS
MONOGASTRIC
ESOPHAGUS
STOMACH
SMALL INTESTINE
APPENDIX (HUMANS)
CECUM (APES, HORSES)
LARGE INTESTINE
ANUS

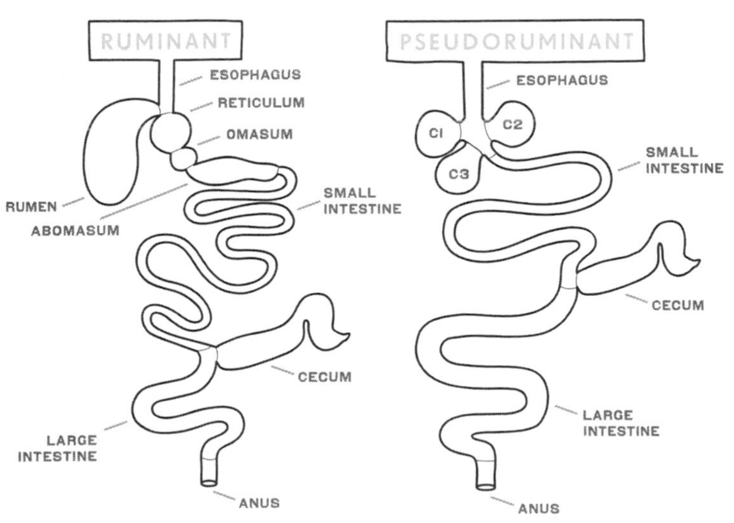
RUMINANT
ESOPHAGUS
RETICULUM
OMASUM
RUMEN
ABOMASUM
SMALL INTESTINE
CECUM
LARGE INTESTINE
ANUS
PSEUDORUMINANT
ESOPHAGUS
C1
C2
C3
SMALL INTESTINE
CECUM
LARGE INTESTINE
ANUS

85 Feed your guts, too

You have about 3 pounds of microscopic, beneficial bacteria and microbes on your skin and in your mouth, lungs, vagina (if you have one), inner mucous regions, and especially in your colon (large intestine). The whole of it is referred to as your microbiome. As host, it's your responsibility to feed it. In exchange for the right kind of food, it will keep you healthy by helping you fight diseases and conditions such as Crohn's, celiac, irritable bowel syndrome, ulcerative colitis, and even yeast infections.

A healthy gut has a large population of these bugs, but when you take antibiotics to kill bad bugs, a lot of good ones get wiped out in the process, and you need to grow more. You do can do that with a fecal transplant—literally having somebody else's poop that's rich in the right kinds of bugs planted into your colon. You can also take a probiotic supplement, but the best way is to eat the right kinds of food—both probiotic (contains the healthy bugs) and prebiotic (provides food for the healthy bugs that are already there). The challenge, easily met, is to eat probiotic, prebiotic, and low carb. Here's a list of foods that work:

Greek yogurt, kefir cheese and any hard cheese including the bacteria-laden veiny blue ones, unpasteurized sauerkraut and pickles, kombucha tea, kimchi, and miso soup. Kefir-the-drink always makes the probiotic team because it's fermented, but it's still too high in carbs for a strict diet. Miso is made from soybeans, but in this form they're fermented and healthier, so in a pinch, go ahead.

Prebiotic foods, which feed good bacteria, include roots and tubers, which tend to be high in carbs; and dark green leaves, which are thankfully low in carbs. (If you have a choice between a sweet potato and Swiss chard, go with the chard.) The bacteria in your colon breaks down the food by fermentation—this is how they "eat" them—just as a cow does in its rumen, and a horse does in its cecum. And a by-product of this digestion-by-fermentation is fatty acids that are used as energy.

Don't take antibiotics "just in case," or at the drop of a hat. They cast a wide net and kill both bad and good bugs, so if you've taken a lot of them, it's especially important to nurture your gut back to health with the right foods. It's easy enough to do this and stay really low-carb.

86 You're technically an omnivore, but your digestive system is 98 percent carnivore

Omni means "all," and omnivores eat and digest all kinds of foods. In our case, we got our omnivorous foundation from our leaf- and fruit-eating ancestors, the apes. An ape can digest tough, chewy leaves and fibrous fruit because, as you now know, it has long intestines and a large cecum to deal with them.

Being omnivorous is a plus when food is scarce, but when food is abundant, it often leads to eating foods that don't kill us immediately, but degrade our health over time, like potatoes, candy, cereal, and soybean oil.

But omnivore or not, for most of the past 2.4 million years we've been eating mostly meat, and have lost the ability to thrive on roughage and plant matter. Mild intolerance makes you fart, but more serious rejection is manifested as gluten intolerance, celiac disease, and Crohn's disease. All are made better by a diet of fully digestible foods that don't pack your guts with undigested plant matter to ferment and feed the bacteria that causes the irritation.

87 Hunger and homeostasis

The hunger you feel as a pang when you haven't eaten for a while is your body telling you it's about out of fuel, so eat. You may think, "Hey, I'm eating plenty, I'm getting fat, I've got too much fuel," but that's only partly true. You have the fuel, but when it's in the form of body fat, you can't access it as energy.

Here's a decent, if not perfect, analogy: You're driving a Ford pickup across Nevada, and—*oh crap!*—your gas tank is almost empty, the car is sputtering, and the nearest Texaco is 75 miles ahead. The irony is that you have 500 gallons of crude oil in 5-gallon jugs in the bed, which might be enough to make 5 day's worth of gas, but you can't refine it into gasoline and burn it up as fuel.

The crude oil in the jugs is the fat on your belly. The crude needs a chemical process to turn it into gas before it can enter your tank and run your car. The belly fat (stored as triglycerides) needs to become fatty acids and get into your blood to make you run without making you fat.

In the car analogy, you're screwed, because you're a car driver, not a mobile oil refiner. In the fat analogy, there's hope, because you're an eater, and when you eat the right foods, the belly fat becomes burnable as fuel, and off it comes.

Insulin in your blood drove the fatty acids into your fat cells and turned them into unburnable triglycerides, and the absence of insulin in your blood will reverse the process.

It really is all about insulin; and when it's all about insulin, it's all about the glucose that drives insulin. And when it's all about glucose, it's all about carbohydrates. The insulin spike from carbohydrates directs glucose beyond your immediate needs to fat creation, and prevents you from burning body fat as fuel. Your body stays hungry as a way to remind you to constantly feed it this inefficient fuel. On a high-carb diet, you're always lethargic (if you try to resist refueling) or hungry.

Cut way, way back on carbs to minimize the amount of insulin going into your blood. Exercise a little to burn off the glucose. The combination of not eating carbs and burning off some glucose through exercise will keep your blood sugar and insulin low enough to allow your body fat to become body fuel. Then good stuff happens.

Without high blood sugar and the resulting high insulin interfering, you'll switch fuels from glucose to fat. As long as you maintain low glucose and insulin—which you do by shunning carbohydrates—your body fat (as triglycerides) will continue to break down into fatty acids and flow off your hips and into your blood, where it becomes your personal fuel, your source of energy, your own gasoline.

In this way, your body burns the calories you've been storing as fat on your hips, belly, and buttocks, unable to burn them as fuel because you've been living with the insulin in your blood (a result of high blood sugar from eating carbs). With a reservoir of fuel so deep and accessible, hunger pangs and urges disappear, you eat less (because you're tapping into your body fat), and you lose weight.

On a super low-carb diet, your caloric demands are being shared by body fat and the food on your plate, so you don't have to eat as much. Your energy supply is constant because it comes from fat and you don't get desperately hungry.

88 Running more on ketones, less on glucose

Since all your cells thrive on glucose and the best dietary source of glucose is carbohydrates, cutting back carbs might seem foolish, even dangerous. It's the opposite. Your prehistoric ancestors lived in carb-scarce times and fueled themselves on fat—the fat they ate and the fat they stored—and they passed on this ability to derive fuel from fat to you.

But carbohydrates screw it up. You get your giddyup from fat—and *burn it off in the process*—only if you create the same internal conditions that your prehistoric ancestors had, and here's how you do that.

For a couple of weeks, eat fewer than 40 grams of carbs a day (a medium banana has 30 grams, a piece of bread has about 22 grams). Forty grams isn't magic; it's just a number that will kick most people into ketosis. Your number could be 60, or it might be 20. During these two weeks, exercise moderately to burn glucose as energy, helping lower the amount in your blood. The goal is to lower your blood glucose to between 65 and 75 milligrams of glucose per deciliter of blood—enough glucose to keep you functioning but not enough to fuel your muscles and organs, so you'll be tapping into your reserve of glucose stored in your liver as glycogen.

Then, when you run out of glycogen (your glucose reserve) your liver will get the signal it needs to replenish glucose and trigger a process called gluconeogenesis—breaking down your muscles to make glucose. At the same time, some of your body fat (stored as triglycerides) breaks down to fatty acids, which flow out of your hips and belly into your blood and then to your muscles, which burn them for fuel. With this new supply of fat-fuel there's less dependence on glucose, so gluconeogenesis stops, and you quit breaking down muscle.

With your glucose levels low but sustainable, and as a by-product of burning fatty acids for energy, your liver begins to make ketone bodies: beta-hydroxybutyrate, acetone, and acetoacetate. These are organic, natural, healthy, beneficial molecules that provide fuel for cells, muscles, and organs when there's no glucose to burn. One of those organs is your brain, the biggest glucose hog in your body. It's typically 2.5 percent of your body weight, but it uses 23 percent of your glucose. Ketones are better brain and body fuel. Training your body to switch fuels from glucose to fat and ketones may seem extreme because you may have to change your diet significantly to make it happen, but remember, it was normal for millions of years. It's the exception now only because we eat so many carbohydrates, which keeps blood sugar too high for ketogenesis (ketone-making).

Just go for it. During the first few weeks of carb restriction, you'll crave them—partly because your body is seeking glucose fuel before it's learned to burn fat, and partly out of habit. When you've had your sacred oatmeal and orange juice for breakfast every day for 20 years, it's hard not to open the cupboard and grab Grandpa Quaker, who was fat himself. But suffer through it, because once you're burning your body fat and making ketones, great things happen:

- You'll burn body fat for fuel instead of packing more of it on your body.
- You won't get nearly as hungry. Your body is consuming its own fat for energy, so your eating urges subside.

- You'll be able to exercise longer on a lot fewer calories. You'll need to stay watered and salted, but when you're burning your own body fat for energy, you won't have to consume as many calories and you won't be hungry. You'll be able to hike, ride a bike, or surf for several hours without replacing the calories you're burning, because you're burning body fat.
- You'll lose weight, and you won't be hungry as often. And when you get hungry, it won't be desperate, light-headed, low-blood-sugar hungry. When you burn fat, your blood sugar level doesn't spike and plummet the way it does when you burn sugar.

Some medical conditions including Type 1 diabetes can make running on ketones risky, so ask your doctor and make sure your doc doesn't confuse ketosis with *ketoacidosis*. Ketosis means you're burning body fat for fuel, sort of a clean energy for your cells—so it's good. Ketoacidosis is when ketones overpopulate your blood and turn it acidic, and it can kill you (so it's bad). Ketoacidosis is a threat only to Type 1 diabetics who don't produce insulin to prevent the overdose. If you're not Type 1, it's not a problem.

In ketosis, you burn body fat instead of making more of it, and to get there—as usual—you need to cut way back on carbs.

89 Cancer thrives on glucose but can't live on ketones

Normal healthy cells need fuel and oxygen, and can run on either oxidized sugar (from carbohydrates) or ketones (from fat). But most cancer cells can make energy only from fermented sugar, and you give them all they need when you eat carbohydrates.

One cancer-fighting strategy is to eat a ketogenic diet, which deprives the cancer of the sugar it needs to grow. Just because cancer thrives on sugar doesn't mean eating bread and fruit causes cancer, or that giving them up will cure it. But cancer cells are such sugar hogs that when doctors suspect you have cancer but don't know exactly where, they identify the cancerous area with a PET scan (positron emission tomography), in which they inject you with a radioactive form of glucose, which leads them to the cancer. Ketogenic diets alone won't vanquish the cancer, but there is compelling evidence that ketogenic diets can contribute to the fight, so discuss them with your oncologist.

There's ongoing research to figure out how to let glucose get to the normal cells but not to the cancer—which would mean you could eat a regular (carb-heavy) diet and still starve the cancer cells. But so far no luck. Until there's a breakthrough, it's at least prudent to minimize the cancer fuel by minimizing carbohydrates.

90 How to make more fat and how to burn it up

There are two forms of fat in your body: triglycerides and fatty acids.

The fat that you eat—the fat in your food—is in the form of triglycerides. Triglyceride molecules are made of three small fatty acid molecules bound to a molecule of glycerol. Your liver makes triglycerides to move fat around in your body, using your bloodstream as a kind of highway. In the liver, triglycerides help form the bad kind of cholesterol (LDL type B) that clogs arteries. And triglycerides in your blood become the fat you pack onto your belly that can't be burned as energy during exercise.

The other kind of fat—that you can burn as energy when you create the right internal conditions—is in a form called fatty acids, which don't pack your arteries or get stored as body fat. Triglycerides can become fatty acids and fatty acids can become triglycerides, and when it comes to losing weight and getting rid of hunger and getting healthy, the whole trick is to convert triglycerides that hurt you to fatty acids that help you. As you're reading this, either triglycerides are breaking down into fatty acids to be burned as energy, making you less fat, or fatty acids are clustering together with glycerol to make more triglycerides for you to store on your waist and make you fatter.

91 Cholesterol, triglycerides, and artery health

Cholesterol is a lipoprotein—a fatty protein that's in all your cells. You can't live without it, but there's good, bad, and neutral cholesterol. HDL (high-density lipoprotein) is good, because it unclogs your arteries. LDL (low-density lipoprotein) is usually branded bad, but that's not fair. It can be either neutral (Pattern A), which is harmless, or bad (Pattern B), the stuff that clogs arteries.

A standard "lipid panel" (blood test) doesn't differentiate between the good and bad LDL, so your LDL score alone doesn't tell much. But there are two scores that do: HDL and triglycerides (TG). TGs deliver the bad kind of LDL into your artery walls. HDL removes it.

If your TGs are four times as high as your HDL (TG 200, HDL 50, for a ratio of 4:1), your arteries are likely in bad shape. A reasonable goal is to get your TG down to 120, and your HDL up to 60—a 2:1 ratio, which is considered safe. If you can get the HDL to 70 and the TG down to 60 or so, you won't be clogging arteries.

To lower your TG, cut back on carbohydrates, because only carbs drive up TG. To raise your HDL, cut out all bad fats (see page 30), eat only good fats (see page 28), and exercise with strain and intensity. This will keep your arteries running clear and clean.

92 Diabetes primer for nondiabetics

There are at least two and arguably three kinds of diabetes.

Type 1 used to be called "childhood diabetes," because it most commonly shows up in children. It's an autoimmune disease—where your body mistakes helpful antibodies for invaders. With no insulin to lower the blood glucose, you'd die of glucose poisoning if you ate carbohydrates. So when type 1 diabetics eat carbohydrates, they take insulin to stay alive. About one in ten diabetics is Type 1.

Type 2 diabetes used to be called "adult-onset diabetes" because it took thirty or more years of bad eating to develop it. Now that kids eat and drink more sugar than ever, they're wearing out their pancreas before adulthood, so now we call it Type 2. In Type 2 diabetes, the pancreas still makes insulin, but the cells reject it, refuse to gobble it up, as though collectively saying, "No, man—we're not going to keep mopping up your mess. We're here for emergencies, not to save you from your addiction to soda and bread, cornflakes and orange juice, sports drinks and energy bars. You obviously don't care, so we're slacking off, too."

Type 2 diabetes often leads to an overproduction of insulin, as if quantity will make up for lack of quality—like fielding a basketball team with eight so-so players instead of five good ones. The insulin, though ineffective in lowering blood sugar, remains supereffective in making a body gain weight. That's why Type 2 diabetics are often fat. Insulin is so effective in making you put on weight that in the 1940s doctors prescribed it for anorexics.

93 Understand and test your own blood sugar

Your fasting blood sugar score is how much sugar is in your blood when you haven't had anything to eat or drink besides water for 8 to 10 hours or so. Measure it in the morning half an hour after you get up, because there's something known as the "morning paradox," where your blood sugar is higher as soon as you wake up than it is a bit later.

Your score is measured in milligrams per deciliter (mg/dl), and healthy is 70 to 90 milligrams, although a more conservative range would take it up to 100. If you live in America and have been eating a low-fat, high-carb diet and have gained 10 or more pounds of fat in the last 20 years, you won't score below 90. An 80 takes effort, know-how, and pretty much no fruit. Below 80 takes real effort, but is a reasonable goal for anybody who's not already diabetic. Many Type 2 diabetics who go hard-core low-carb can score in the mid-80s.

If it was 1961 and you wanted to measure your blood sugar at home, the 3-pound test meter would set you back $650 and you'd still need a doctor's prescription to buy it. You might have been arrested if you were caught with one without a note from your doctor. Today's meters weigh an ounce or two, cost less than $25, and due to the epidemic of Type 2 diabetes, every pharmacy in the country sells them cheap two aisles down from the lipstick.

The One-Touch Ultra-Mini is the Toyota Camry/ Parker Jotter/ Ray-Ban Wayfarer of glucose meters—good enough for any purpose. You can buy the strips cheap online, or get them from the pharmacist.

Read the instructions, but here's the procedure:

1 Get up in the morning, sit around for half an hour, then wash your hands.

2 Stick a test strip in the meter and wait 2 seconds for the "ready to accept blood" signal.

3 Prick yourself. A spring-loaded needle takes the bravery out of the prick.

4 Squeeze a drop of blood onto the strip and wait 5 seconds for your score.

A score in high 90s won't concern a doctor used to seeing blind, diabetic amputees, but it's on the high side of normal, and with no change in diet, it'll grow to 105, 110 in a few years, higher after that. If your fasting blood glucose score is 120 mg/dl or higher now, go to your doctor and request an A1C test, which gives your average glucose score for the past three months, in millimoles. To convert millimoles (mM) to mg/dl so you can compare it to your random, fasting glucose score, multiply them by 18. For instance, an A1C score of 5.7 mM equates to an average glucose score of 103.5 mg/dl, which won't freak out a doctor, but is a sign that you've taken a wrong turn and are now on the the long road to weight gain and maybe diabetes. Cut the carbs and get it down to the mid-80s or below. You'll shed fat and stay far away from diabetes.

94 In for a penny, in for a pound: Test your ketones, too

Once you're used to testing your glucose, testing your ketone production—to verify whether or not you're burning body fat—is just a hop, step, and a jump away. If you haven't tested either yet, the prospect of testing your blood ketones may seem like a dark, weird thing to do, but that's the wrong way to think about it. Technology makes it possible to self-test at home, and it's an easy way to learn something that just a few decades ago not even the Mayo Clinic could tell you. Just do it.

In ketosis, you're powering your personal machine on body fat, and getting leaner as you go. Since your body is getting calories from its stored fat, it doesn't demand that you eat so much, so often. Most people in ketosis do fine on one main meal a day and a few fatty snacks. A fatty drink for breakfast; a small hunk of cheese with macadamia nuts for brunch; late lunch of Greek yogurt and either more cheese, macadamias, or half a can of salmon; dinner is a salad with an omelet; late-night snack is fatty tea with a few macadamias, Greek yogurt, or cheese.

A ketosis naysayer will point out that the calories add up to less than 1,500 so it's the calories that get the credit for weight loss, not the ketosis. Here's what you say to that: "It may be only 1,500 calories, but I'm *full* on those 1,500 because the other 2,000 or so calories I need for the day are coming from body fat. If I were to eat only 1,500 carb-ish calories, I'd be starving and miserable." It is true.

There are three ways to measure your ketone levels.

1 THE INEXPENSIVE BUT INACCURATE WAY

Small strips ("Ketostix" is one brand) that you either pee on or dip into pee. All pharmacies have them, but they don't measure beta-hydroxybutyrate, the most stable and easily measured ketone body. They cost less than $1 each, but you have to buy about 20 at a time, and that's a lot to spend for inaccurate scores.

2 BREATH TESTER

It measures exhaled acetone (a ketone). These widgets sell for about $100 or a bit more, but should appeal to those who don't like to prick themselves, and cost less per test than the following method.

3 THE FAR MORE ACCURATE AND NOT-THAT-EXPENSIVE WAY

Blood testing is the way to go. Ketone blood testing is a lot like glucose testing, with its own meter and strips. The Abbott Precision Xtra blood ketone monitor is the meter of choice. Pharmacies don't always stock the test strips, but you can get them online. Canadadrugs.com has them for as low as $3 each, when you buy them online from Canada.

The scores are in millimoles, and the numbers to look for are between 0.5 and 5.0. The 0.5 indicates you're just barely in ketosis. It'll take some effort to get there, and you'll go through a dozen or more $3 strips showing you at 0.2 to 0.3 before your first 0.5.

To get scores between 0.5 and 5 takes a combination of super low-carb eating, skipping a meal now and then, and plenty of exercise. A score of 3.5 indicates lots of fat burning. Unless you're a Type 1 diabetic, you won't go dangerously above 5.0, and in fact, may never even reach 3.0.

If you're curious about your ketone levels but you don't want to test them, extrapolate from your fasting glucose score. For most people, blood glucose levels of 75 or less are too low to supply energy for exercise, so your body will turn to stores of body fat instead, and produce ketones in the process.

95 Is your spit making you fat?

No, your spit isn't making you fat, but it may be making it harder for you to lose it. Going back far enough, we're all the product of the same evolution, but certain ethnicities are less carbohydrate tolerant than others because they have less amylase in their spit.

Amylase is an enzyme that predigests starch while it's still in your mouth, effectively reducing the sugar load, so by the time the carbs get to your intestines and the glucose starts invading your blood, there's less of it. Less glucose means less insulin, less fat storage, less chance of getting diabetes, and better health in general.

How much amylase you have in your spit is related to how long your genes have had to adapt to carbohydrates. If your ancestors got in on the agricultural revolution when it began about 12,000 years ago in what's now the Middle East, they probably evolved to have more amylase and have passed the advantage on to you. That doesn't make you fat-proof—you can still blow out your pancreas with decades of carbs—but it can cut back the glucose response by up to 10 percent, a huge starting advantage.

On the other end of the amylase-in-spit spectrum are Africans, Hispanics, and Native Americans, all of whom have had much shorter exposure to high-carb diets and tend to have the lowest concentrations of amylase in their spit, making it harder for them to stay slender and avoid diabetes if they're eating a lot of carbs.

You've probably heard of Dr. Oz. He's from Turkey, due north of what used to be Phoenicia, smack dab in the Middle East, the birthplace of the agricultural revolution, where grains were first cultivated. Dr. Oz is skinny and counsels people on what to eat. For years, he has recommended low-fat diets that are inevitably high carb, which is understandable, because that's what works for him. But being Turkish, Dr. Oz likely has high-amylase spit, which gives him an advantage other people might not have.

Oprah is a big fan of Oz, but she probably has less amylase in her spit than Dr. Oz does, so she'll find it harder to lose weight on quinoa and fresh fruit. If Oprah were from Turkey and Oz were from Africa, she might be the wispy one. As it is, Oprah's best chance of losing weight is a super low-carb, ketogenic diet.

Weight management is complex and involves genetics, diet, exercise, culture, social pressures, and commercial influence. But when all else is equal, people with more amylase in their spit have an advantage.

96 Alzheimer's: diabetes of the brain?

There are genetic factors that make Alzheimer's disease more likely for some people. Bumps on the head and food additives have been implicated, too. But in 2005, Dr. Suzanne de la Monte and her team at Brown University, curious as to why Type 2 diabetics get Alzheimer's at double the rate of the nondiabetic population, discovered that a lot of the traits of Alzheimer's disease in the brain are caused by insulin resistance.

Ordinarily, your brain uses about 23 percent of your glucose. But when the brain cells (neurons) become insulin-resistant, they die, and when enough die, you get Alzheimer's. Is this a simplification? Of course. This is not a textbook. But that's basically what happens. The insulin-resistance is so similar (just in a different part of the body) that Dr. de la Monte suggested Alzheimer's could be called Type 3 diabetes.

The treatments are similar, too. In both cases, when glucose is not fueling the cells, ketones can do the job, and in the case of Alzheimer's, one treatment, which shows good results in arresting and even reversing some of the symptoms, is coconut oil. Coconut oil is two-thirds medium-chain triglycerides (MCTs), which, when they're metabolized, produce more ketones than other fats do. The ketones supply energy to the neurons when glucose is unavailable, so they stay alive and healthy. But ketones don't automatically contribute just because the cells are hungry for fuel. You have to create the internal conditions that produce ketones. You have to dramatically lower your blood sugar and go into ketosis, and currently the best way to do that is by eating a super low-carb, ketogenic diet, high in medium-chain triglycerides. You get them from pure MCT oil or coconut oil.

Being in ketosis can't undo advanced Alzheimer's, but there is strong evidence that in many cases fueling your neurons with ketones instead of trying in vain to stuff them full of glucose can slow the progression of brain damage, and even reverse it to some degree. If Alzheimer's is part of your life, or you suspect it will be, it will be worth your time to read the article on the National Institutes of Health website, or you can look up "Dr. de la Monte, Type 3 diabetes" on the Internet. The article is technical, but the important information jumps out at you—that the neuron-protecting qualities of ketones (and a ketogenic diet) have been proven therapeutic for many neuro-degenerative disease. Any specialist in the disease can tell you more.

97 A survey isn't a study, a correlation isn't a cause, and an observation is just somebody looking at something

The worst scientists gather data and look for correlations—like when A goes up, B tends to go up, and therefore they conclude and announce that A causes B to rise. They write it up as a study and forward it to the local news team, who presents it as a revelation and delivers it as a sensationalized sound bite of life-changing information. Reporters often have no science background, and in any case are pressured to be first or early with medical discoveries, so they report correlations as facts, and that's the problem.

Correlational "studies" like this have convinced most of the country that red meat is bad and whole grains are good. But these claims don't consider that, hey, with all the anti–red meat and pro–whole grain noise out there, it's possible that those who eat red meat in spite of that just might thumb their nose at every bit of health advice (including the good) that comes their way. They might be among the "screw it, I'll eat and drink whatever I want!" crowd. To extend that idea, people who go out of their way to eat brown rice and whole-wheat pasta probably also don't smoke, do wear sunscreen in the desert and in the mountains, and avoid skin contact with known toxins. These are contributing factors (independent variables, in science terms) that can't be counted in a correlational "study."

It's hard, expensive, usually impractical, often impossible to conduct a rigorous double-blind study of the effect of diet on humans, because rigorousness requires both a large sample of subjects for a year or more (impractical and expensive when you have to pay them) and a nearly identical biology (basically impossible even with the closest lab tests). That's why most scientific studies are on rodents and fruit flies: Their habits and generational histories can be controlled. But when the study is something like the effect of meat on health, and the test subjects are animals that have not evolved to digest meat, the conclusions have to be suspect. One recently formed organization founded and funded to conduct the most rigorous, objective studies on diet and health is the Nutrition Science Initiative (nusi.org).

Dietary health is never as simple as Cabbage Equals Health and Beef Equals Cancer, but people like simple solutions to complex problems, and the easier the sound bite is to remember, the more likely it is to guide food choices. But even amid all the bad science and nonsense food advice out there, there is a clear trend toward reducing carbs and sugar—inevitable, since this is the path that works.

WHAT TO THINK ABOUT NOW

This part of the book leans toward the philosophical, which is just a way of saying there are unresolved issues here, reasonable people will disagree, and this is just what I think. If you disagree with something (you will), I hope it won't make you throw down the book, disregard everything, and eat a big plate of pasta with a side of bread, washed down with apple juice.

98 You can be fat and happy, but can you be fat and healthy?

There's a well-meaning movement to encourage you to accept your excess fat—to embrace it, call it beautiful, say it's sexy. It can be those things, but the eagerness to be OK with being fat is based on the myth that there's no connection between outer appearance and inner health, that you can simply eat too many calories and store them as fat and still be perfectly healthy inside, with killer blood scores and arteries as clean as PVC pipes fresh from the hardware store.

You *can't* gain a lot of weight on the outside and be healthy on the inside, because the same things that make you fat also raise your risk for high blood pressure, diabetes, heart disease, cancer, and Alzheimer's. You can walk around saying, "I feel great!", but your insides will eventually catch up to your outsides. If you're fat and don't have any diseases or symptoms, you're lucky, but you might be on your way, and you should think of your excess fat as a warning of worse things to come if you don't change course.

If there were truly no hope of losing fat, you'd be better off accepting it than beating yourself up about it. But most fat is a result of the carbohydrates–blood sugar–insulin and insulin-resistance progression, and the solution could be as easy as eating the bacon and eggs, and leaving behind the whole-wheat toast and orange juice.

99 If your child is overweight

It's hard to see your children pay the social costs of being heavy, but it's even harder to discuss it with them. Many parents avoid the awkward, possibly damaging talk, but these tips might help:

- **DON'T KEEP CARBS IN THE HOUSE.** Even skinny people are better off without carbs, and if nobody's eating them it'll be easier for your overweight child to refrain. Breakfast is the most harried meal in most homes, but eggs take 5 minutes and Greek yogurt takes 30 seconds. You won't have this control outside the home, but healthy practices at home may rub off. If skinny siblings squawk, have a talk about "family."
- **TURN SHAME TO BLAME.** Most kids feel some sense of shame for being overweight. It's misplaced. Most weight problems are caused by following bad advice, so you and they should blame the bad advisers—the advertisers, medical community, and nutrition experts who tout low-fat foods, lots of exercise, and calorie counting as a way to lose weight.
- **TEACH THEM ABOUT CARBS** and come up with creative alternatives. Some of the recipes that follow will prove that foods can taste as good or better without carbs.
- **DON'T RULE OUT MEASURING BLOOD SUGAR** scores and charting them as a sign of progress. Blood sugar scores are a more visible sign of improvement than a pound or two of weight loss.

100 Have you ever followed bad advice?

Sometimes people who don't have a weight problem look at people who do and think they don't care, have just given up, or choose not to change. They think, *Why did you keep doing what you were doing when you'd gained 50 pounds? You must have noticed, so why did you keep eating that stuff?*

If you're fat, you know you're not lazy, gluttonous, or indifferent. You've just been following the advice of doctors, nutritionists, authors, skinny friends, personal trainers, magazines, and favorite celebrities who all say the same thing: exercise more, eat fewer calories, eat more complex carbs, eat less fat, go for the fresh fruit and whole grains. But you keep gaining, and you're starting to accept this as your fate: This is *the way you are* now.

Quit following the bad advice. Eat fat to fill you up, cut way back on carbs so you don't raise your insulin and create your own constant hunger and fat storage. Test your glucose, test your ketones, find out what the food you eat is doing to your insides. Most likely, it's spiking your blood sugar and insulin.

101 Pros and cons of being a teenage eater

- **PROS:** You'll never build muscle faster than you will now, when you're growing and have naturally high levels of growth hormone to take advantage of. You'll get more dramatic results and faster results than adults do, with less effort—but you have to try a little: You have to put in that 3 to 7 minutes a day. Get strong now, and establish a personal standard that makes health and strength normal, and makes maintaining it for the rest of your life relatively easy.
- **CONS:** You'll get faulty feedback, and are likely to form bad habits, which by the time you're in your thirties will make you fat and unhealthy. If you live on carbs now but aren't fat, it's likely due to a combination of insulin-sensitivity (you haven't worn out your pancreas yet) and growth hormone (testosterone for boys). Both are peaking and make it easy for you to stay lean and build muscle.

Your levels of growth hormone decline as you age, though, and by your late thirties, you'll find yourself losing muscle and gaining fat.

If you're a teenager, take advantage of your raging hormones and cut way back on carbs so you don't continue to require more and more insulin for a given load of carbs as you age—making you fatter every year. Be one of the rare old people who find it easy to stay lean.

102 Recalibrate your taste buds

If you've eaten out a lot in good restaurants and there's a good cook at home, chances are your palate has gotten pickier over the years, and now you turn up your nose at meals hobos would tussle over. Have you become a taste wimp? Here's a test:

- Do you eat eggplant only as eggplant Parmesan, and not sliced and steamed or fried with minimal seasoning?
- Do you eat restaurant salmon but never salmon out of the can?
- Do you eat sardines, ever?
- Do you say "I love Brussels sprouts!" but eat them only slathered in butter, garlic, and cheese?

Professional chefs and gourmet cooks rely on your refined palate, but there's nothing wrong with stretching it downward a bit. It won't stop you from liking or appreciating the tastiest foods; it'll just help you like some healthy foods you can barely tolerate now and tolerate foods that right now you can't stand.

To recalibrate, start with foods just slightly out of reach, seasoned less than you prefer, cooked a different way, swimming in less sweet and spicy sauce. If they're plants, try steamed rather than sautéed, or raw rather than cooked. If it's meat, forget the sugary marinade and barbecue sauce.

103 Cats and dogs are carnivores, so feed them carne

Most dog and cat foods are cheapened with carbohydrates—which is why there are so many fat pets that they have their own fat camps now. You can get grain-free pet food, but you still have to read the labels: One of the better and more expensive brands still has tomatoes, blueberries, apples, broccoli, spinach, parsley, flaxseed, peas, kale, and three kinds of potatoes—all are foods to win the hearts of dog owners, but wrong for dogs.

It's better to just serve yourself more steak or bacon than you need and skim some off for the dog. When you want four eggs with cheese, fry up five and give Bowser the spare. Or buy cheap one-pound cans of salmon or mackerel, and make that the go-to dog or cat food. Throw in a pet multivitamin if it makes you feel better, but they'll do fine without it. Don't feed Spuds McKenzie spuds, feed him other animals.

It's a win-win-win. The feces of meat-eating dogs doesn't stink as much as the feces from grain-eating dogs. And people on low-carb diets don't produce as much gas. It's healthier and less smelly all around.

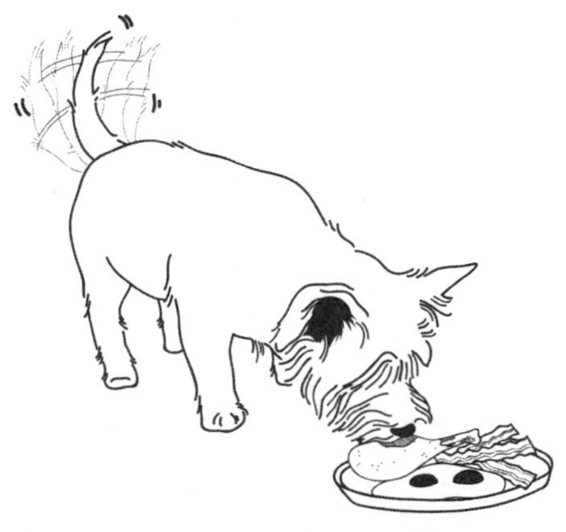

104 Bad advice from the pros

Many of the organizations that by their name and influence suggest expertise and authority on matters of health—diabetes or heart disease especially—continue to give bad advice. One of these organizations, the American Diabetes Association, tells diabetics to eat about 200 grams of carbs per day, 50 to 75 grams of carbs per meal, to get half their calories from carbs. Any diabetic who follows that advice will require regular doses of insulin to lower the blood sugar spikes from the carbs, will find it impossible to lose weight, and is assured a future that includes at least some of the problems related to diabetes—bad circulation, slow healing, impotence, inability to walk, blindness, and Alzheimer's.

By the time you have Type 2 diabetes, you've already eaten 90 percent of your life's allotment of carbs. You've worn out your pancreas and made carbs poison to you. The diabetes organizations and media tell you to avoid Coke and go moderate on the sweets (and take your insulin), but that just slows the decline. Nondiabetics get to nibble on bread, but you shouldn't. When you're a Type-2 diabetic, limiting your carbs to 30 grams a day is much better advice. It will reduce and maybe even eliminate your need for insulin, and your health will improve dramatically. When you already have Type 2 diabetes, the moderation ship has sailed.

When the topic is weight gain and cardiovascular health, almost every major, national, well-established health care organization or academic institution advises you to eat the opposite of what I recommend. Intuitively, it makes sense that eating less fat would make you and your arteries less fat, so that's an easy sell even though it's not true. The counterintuitive truth that you have to gobble up fat to lose fat and clear out your arteries is a harder sell, because it requires an understanding of blood sugar, insulin, fat creation and storage, and homeostastis. But any doctor, neighbor, or governmental organization that continues to espouse high-carb, low-fat diets for health is wrong, and in time this will be common knowledge. When your diet is dominated by healthy fats and you limit carbohydrates to less than 50 grams per day—or if you're already diabetic, maybe 30 grams per day or less—you'll notice a dramatic improvement in your shape and health.

105 When animals are available, eat them

Eating animals isn't an option for the whole world. There are too many people and not enough animals. But just because it won't work for the whole world is no reason to limit yourself to plants, or to feel guilty about eating animals. Let that whole-world standard shame you every time you drive your car or fly in a plane, or for every pair of leather shoes you buy just for pleasure. But don't listen to it when it comes to feeding your body the food it needs to be healthy.

Besides, all eating involves some kind of death. Tilling land for corn, rice, and soybeans alters the natural ecosystem and kills many of the plants and animals that depend on it, all so people can prepare the acreage for a specific crop that in most cases they shouldn't be eating in the first place.

Eating animals isn't totally clean, either, but there are ways to grow and get food that minimize the toll on the environment and the suffering of the animals. Hunting and fishing locally is the winner, but that's not practical for the majority, so at least shop with a conscience. However you obtain your animals, the better health that comes of eating them will make you less likely to need medicine, hospitalization, special procedures, or skilled nursing later on. Everybody benefits when you can manage your own tasks as you age, and a high-fat, super low-carbohydrate diet makes that more likely.

106 Don't let the clock be the boss of your piehole

Even when you do everything right and you're in ketosis a lot of the time, there's still the pull of having to eat when everybody else is eating, getting three squares a day with the classic breakfast, lunch, and dinner. But once you're burning fat for calories, you won't need more than one main meal a day. Then, if you feel like eating with everyone else, eat fatty snacks—cheese, macadamias, or low-carb chocolate. Instead of chips, eat seaweed squares (see "Recalibrate your taste buds," on page 182). Until you experience it, it's hard to imagine not being hungry when you haven't eaten for 6 hours, but on a high-fat, super low-carb diet that has you burning body fat for fuel, you won't be.

If you have a family, eat social dinners and talk to one another. There are more things in life than getting ripped, and eating together is one of them, so don't be an outcast (but also, don't eat the pasta). When you're on your own, though, make your meals need-based, not clock-based. You'll find it's easy to get down to ten main meals a week, with small fatty snacks to fill in the gaps, as your stomach takes control.

RECIPES

Even an oaf can make things taste good with sugar and flour, but knowing about blood sugar and insulin makes it hard to enjoy them. If you have learned about insulin's role in getting fat by reading this book, then the recipes that follow may be consolation for your new eating program. If these recipes are not to your taste or not fancy enough, look up the dozens of good low-carb cookbooks out there. Some of mine were inspired by already published recipes, but I've changed them to suit my taste, and in doing so, I cut out even more of the carbs.

Fantastic fake pancakes

The pancakes come out thin, like crêpes, and are *better* than real pancakes. Make them for your high-carbin' friends and guests and serve them with actual maple syrup. But on the ones you serve yourself, use butter, ghee, or blueberries. SERVES 1 OR 2

- 4 eggs
- 4 ounces cream cheese, at room temperature
- 2 teaspoons ground flaxseed meal
- 2 teaspoons ground cinnamon
- 1 tablespoon butter or ghee, for frying and serving
- Maple syrup, for serving

PREHEAT the oven to 200°F. Place a large platter in the oven to warm.

IN A LARGE BOWL, lightly beat the eggs. Add the cream cheese, flaxseed meal, and cinnamon, and stir to combine well.

IN A LARGE SKILLET over medium-high heat, melt the butter or ghee, and swirl it around to coat the bottom of the pan.

WHEN the pan is quite hot, pour three or four scoops of batter into the pan to make pancakes about the diameter of an orange. They'll be easier to turn than big pancakes.

COOK on one side until bubbles form on top and the underside is browned, about 1½ minutes. Flip them over, and cook the other side for about 1 more minute. Remove to the plate in the oven to keep them warm until you've cooked all the pancakes. Add more butter or ghee to the pan for each batch, as needed.

SERVE hot or cold.

Fake pizza with no crust

Eggplant is the violator of the "only green vegetables" rule, but it's low in carbs, and, being a cellulose-based vegetable, you won't thoroughly digest them all. This fake pizza is as good as real. SERVES 4

- Butter, for greasing the baking dish
- One 1½-pound eggplant, cut into ¼-inch-thick slices
- 2 cups shredded mozzarella cheese
- 1 cup shredded Parmesan cheese
- 1 cup spaghetti sauce (with no added sugar)
- 1 teaspoon dried basil
- 1 teaspoon dried oregano
- 1 teaspoon dried Italian seasoning

PREHEAT the oven to 375°F. Lightly butter a 9-by-12-inch glass or ceramic baking dish.

OVERLAP half of the eggplant slices to form a layer in the prepared baking dish. Sprinkle on ¾ cup of the mozzarella, ½ cup of the Parmesan, and spoon on ¾ cup of the sauce. Sprinkle on ½ teaspoon each of the basil, oregano, and Italian seasoning. For a second layer, add the remaining half of the eggplant, and sprinkle with ¾ cup of the mozzarella, ½ cup of the Parmesan, ¼ cup of the sauce, and ½ teaspoon each of the basil, oregano, and Italian seasoning.

COVER the baking dish snugly with aluminum foil and bake for 40 minutes. Uncover, sprinkle on the remaining ½ cup of the mozzarella, reduce the oven to 350°F, and bake until the cheese has melted, about 5 more minutes.

PLACE the fake pizza on a cooling rack for 10 minutes before cutting into servings. Serve hot.

Fantastic fake quiche

This is as good as the pizza and is even better the second day, cold. The worst thing in it—from an ultra-hard-core, low-carb perspective—is the spinach or broccoli; and when that's the case, you know it's healthy. SERVES 4

- 1 tablespoon butter or ghee
- 1 onion, chopped
- 1 red bell pepper, seeded and chopped (optional)
- One (10-ounce) pkg frozen spinach, defrosted and water squeezed out, or 1 head broccoli cut into small florets
- 6 eggs, lightly beaten
- 3 cups shredded cheese (Havarti, Munster, Cheddar, or Parmesan are all good choices, and can be used in combination)
- 1/4 teaspoon salt
- 1/8 teaspoon pepper

PREHEAT the oven to 350°F. Grease a 9-inch pie pan with butter or ghee.

IN A LARGE SKILLET over medium-high heat, heat the butter or ghee. Add the onion and sauté, stirring often, until soft, about 8 minutes. Add the bell pepper (if using) and cook, stirring often, until tender, about 5 minutes. Add the spinach or broccoli and cook, stirring to combine, until warmed through, about 2 minutes. Remove from the heat.

MIX the eggs, cheese, salt, and pepper in a large bowl, combining well. Stir in the vegetables.

ADD the egg-vegetable mixture to the prepared pie pan and bake for about 40 minutes.

LET the fake quiche cool on a rack for about 10 minutes before cutting. Serve hot, warm, or at room temperature.

Green soup

This is another recipe that will score solid tens across the board, even with bread-eaters. SERVES 6

- 1 tablespoon butter or olive oil
- 1 large onion, chopped
- 2 cloves garlic, finely chopped
- 3 cups vegetable or chicken stock
- 3 medium zucchini, cut into thin slices
- 2 heads (3/4 lb) broccoli, finely chopped
- 1/4 cup heavy cream
- Salt
- Pepper

Pesto

- 2 cups fresh basil leaves
- 1/2 cup shredded Parmesan cheese
- 3 tablespoons pine nuts
- 1/4 cup olive oil
- Salt

HEAT the butter or olive oil in a large skillet over medium-high heat. Add the onion and garlic and sauté, stirring often, until soft, about 5 minutes. Remove from the heat.

IN A LARGE SAUCEPAN over high heat, add the stock and cook until it comes to a boil. Add the zucchini, broccoli, onion, and garlic. Bring back to a boil, then reduce heat to medium and simmer until the zucchini is tender, about 10 minutes. Remove from the heat.

To make the pesto:

IN A BLENDER or food processor, add the basil, Parmesan, pine nuts, olive oil, and season with salt. Blend until smooth. Pour into a medium bowl. Rinse the blender bowl.

TRANSFER the zucchini mixture to the blender or food processor in batches and blend until smooth.

Return the mixture to the saucepan over medium heat. Stir in the cream and 3 tablespoons of pesto. Season with salt and pepper and reheat.

PUT the remaining pesto in a small serving bowl. Serve the soup hot in soup bowls, and pass the pesto for people to help themselves.

Real ratatouille

Ratatouille tastes even better the next day. It can be stored in the refrigerator for up to a week. Serve it at any temperature you like—hot, cold, room temp, or microwaved. And don't hesitate to mix in cheese, eggs, or meat. SERVES 6 TO 8

- 2 large eggplants
- 2 yellow onions
- 3 green bell peppers
- 6 to 8 medium zucchini or summer squash
- 4 large or 8 small tomatoes
- Salt
- 2 to 4 cloves garlic, minced
- Butter, ghee, olive oil, or macadamia nut oil (any and all, for fat)
- 2 bay leaves
- 3 to 4 sprigs thyme
- Pepper
- ½ cup loosely packed thinly sliced basil leaves

CUT the eggplant, onions, bell peppers, zucchini or squash, and tomatoes into bite-size chunks, and put each vegetable in a separate medium bowl.

PUT the eggplant in a colander and toss it with 1 tablespoon salt. Let it sweat in the sink while you prep the other ingredients.

HEAT 1 tablespoon fat in a large soup pot over medium-high heat. Add the onions and a generous pinch of salt and sauté, stirring frequently, until the onions begin to soften, about 4 mintues. Add the bell peppers and cook until they begin to soften, another 4 minutes. Remove to a large bowl.

ADD 2 tablespoons fat to the soup pot over medium-high heat and add the zucchini and a generous pinch of salt. Sauté until the zucchini starts to brown, then remove it to the large bowl.

RINSE the eggplant under running water, squeeze the water out, and put it in a medium bowl. Heat 2 teaspoons fat in a large skillet over medium-high heat, and add the eggplant. Sauté, stirring frequently, until translucent, about 10 minutes. Remove to the large bowl with the other vegetables.

ADD 1 teaspoon fat to the large skillet over low heat, add the garlic, and sauté until it's golden brown, stirring constantly, about 1 minute. Stir in the tomatoes, bay leaves, and thyme sprigs.

ADD the cooked vegetables back into the large skillet and mix evenly. Season with salt and pepper. Simmer, stirring occasionally. Cook for 30 to 45 minutes, if you like the vegetables to remain distinct pieces, or up to 2 hours, if you want it to be mushy, like classic ratatouille. Remove the bay leaves and thyme sprigs and discard. Stir in the basil, and remove from the heat.

SERVE hot or cold.

Diabetes-safe croutons

These uncubed, nontraditional croutons will be the best you've ever tasted, and they won't jack up your blood sugar. MAKES 2 CUPS (ENOUGH FOR A FOUR-SERVING SALAD)

Butter or ghee

2 cups of shredded hard cheese (like Parmesan, Romano, or Cheddar)

PREHEAT the oven to 400°F. Grease an 8-by-8-inch baking pan with butter or ghee.

IN THE PREPARED baking pan, spread out the cheese in an even layer.

BAKE for about 18 minutes. The cheese will melt, forming a thin layer. If you burn it a little, it will be extra good. There's a wide range of acceptability in the cooking of these, and after one batch, you'll know what you want to do next time. When it cools, break it up into "croutons."

Super white "cereal"

Part of the fun of cereal is spooning it into your mouth. This allows that, without the blood sugar effect that comes with that stuff in the box. SERVES 1

- **2/3 cup unsweetened coconut flakes or shredded coconut**
- **1/4 cup unsweetened coconut milk**
- **1 to 2 tablespoons plain unsweetened Greek yogurt**
- **A fistful of macadamia nuts**
- **1/4 cup berries (optional)**
- **1 teaspoon stevia, xylitol, or Truvia (optional)**

PUT the coconut flakes, coconut milk, yogurt, macadamia nuts, berries (if using) in a large cereal bowl, and sprinkle with stevia or Truvia (if using). Dig in!

Fun with cream

When you eat low-carb, you get to eat high-fat, and that means guilt-free cream. Get creative. Here's a start. MAKES ABOUT 2 CUPS

½ pint (1 cup) chilled heavy whipping cream

3 to 6 drops stevia, or 1 teaspoon NuStevia powder, or your favorite nonsugar sweetener

POUR the cream and sweetener into a lidded jar that holds two or three times that volume.

PUT the lid on tightly and shake the jar like a demon for 3 to 7 minutes until the cream thickens. Near the end the shaking will get quieter as the cream thickens, and it's fully whipped cream when it shakes silently. Then, if you keep shaking it, you'll get butter, but the point here is thick, forkable cream, so stop when it's quiet.

NEWS FLASH: It has come to my attention that you can use an electric beater and a medium chilled bowl to make whipped cream fluffier and faster. Apparently this technology has been around for more than half a century and it results in fluffier whipped cream.

TRY a spoonful immediately, then freeze it solid, and eat it colder and thicker the next day.

The chocolate mousse alternative:

ADD 2 tablespoons of unsweetened cocoa powder per half pint (1 cup) of heavy cream. It gets thicker faster with the cocoa powder. Add some sweetener, because the cocoa powder is bitter by itself. If you want your family to like it, you may have to sweeten it.

Chocoroons

I love macaroons, and didn't want to give them up, so I came up with this recipe. Leave out the cocoa powder if you want them white. MAKES 48 CHOCOROONS

- 6 eggs, at room temperature (if they're cold, put them in a bowl and run warm water over them for a minute)
- 1¼ cups fat—roughly half coconut oil and half ghee or butter
- ¾ teaspoon vanilla
- 3 cups shredded unsweetened raw coconut
- 1¼ tablespoons NuStevia or other carbless sweetener (optional)
- ½ teaspoon salt
- 2 tablespoons chia seeds
- 2 tablespoons unsweetened cocoa powder (optional)
- Macadamias to taste or budget

PREHEAT the oven to 350°F. Butter or coconut-spray a baking sheet.

SEPARATE the egg whites and put them into a large bowl. Whip the whites for 3 to 5 minutes. Add the vanilla and mix it in.

MIX the dry ingredients.

MICROWAVE the coconut oil for a minute (or melt it on the stovetop). Melt the ghee or butter the same way, and combine. Add the vanilla.

POUR the liquid fat and egg whites into the bowl with the dry mix and stir it well. Pour it onto a greased baking pan and bake for 18 minutes. Cut into squares while warm.

Coconut butter

Making your own coconut butter is easy, and it's a good thing to know how to do when you run out of your store-bought. This recipe comes with delicious options. MAKES ABOUT 1½ POUNDS

1 pound unsweetened shredded coconut or coconut flakes

¼ cup unsweetened cocoa powder

1 tablespoon stevia or erythritol sweetener or a mix of the two

¼ cup almonds, almond butter, or macadamia nuts

¼ cup finely ground coffee

POUR about three-fourths of the coconut flakes into a food processor or blender, and blend until the coconut becomes a creamy, textured, thick liquid, in 7 to 12 minutes. If the whirring blades force the mix to the side and end up spinning in air, add the remaining coconut to encourage blending. If it's blending just fine, add the rest anyway.

THEN, you can also add any combination of the following, with delicious results: the cocoa powder, stevia, almonds, coffee.

EAT a few spoonfuls while it's still warm from mixing. Pour it into a pan, tubs, or ice cube trays and refrigerate or freeze.

Blue cheese and cherry tomato soup

On a hot day when you're hungry, it's hard to beat this—if you're among the one-in-three who love blue cheese. SERVES 4

3 cups coconut milk

1½ cups shredded unsweetened coconut

4 ounces blue cheese chunks

1½ cups cherry tomatoes

IN A BLENDER or food processor, add the coconut milk, coconut, and blue cheese. Blend until well combined and thick.

PUT the tomatoes in a medium bowl, and pour the coconut–blue cheese mixture over the tomatoes. Eat it with a spoon.

IF YOU LET IT sit overnight in the refrigerator, it will thicken. If you want it really thick, freeze it and eat it like ice cream, but in that case, leave out the cherry tomatoes.

Fantastic blue cheese dressing

The problem with most commercial blue cheese dressings is the cheap, unhealthy, or iffy-at-best oil they contain. Seed oil, almost always. The recipe here doesn't contain oil, but I'm not trying to be low-fat with it, and you can add macadamia or olive oil if you like (try ¼ cup). But it doesn't need it for thickness or smoothness, and if it's not as pourable, so what? The best blue cheese dressings are always the chunkiest ones, anyway. MAKES ABOUT 2¼ CUPS

1 cup plain unsweetened Greek yogurt

1 cup blue cheese crumbles

½ cup plain unsweetened coconut milk

PUT the yogurt, blue cheese, and coconut milk in a blender or food processor. Blend until smooth.

STORE the dressing in the refrigerator in an airtight container for up to 1 week.

Japaneasy soup

What makes this soup so healthy? The salmon has protein and omega-3 fats. The seaweeds have iodine, which is great brain food. The coconut oil is ⅔ medium-chain triglycerides, which are not stored as fat, and produce more ketones than any other form of fat. The butter or ghee tastes good and does no harm. The vegetables are largely harmless filler, but if you cut them fine, more vitamins will leach out into the water, where they're more digestible. The bone stock jacks up the magnesium. Eggs add fat, protein, and a little familiarity.

Nori is Japanese dried seaweed made into sheets. For the nori, get the expensive kind with nothing added. Kombu is Japanese thick dried seaweed made into sticks. The kombu instructions may say to remove it after it's leaked some of the good stuff into the water. I like to keep it in there and eat it. It's bland, chewy, and it comes from the sea, so my guess is it's good for you. SERVES 4

1 quart chicken or beef bone low-sodium stock

Kombu, broken into 24 or more bite-size pieces

1 bunch (about 3 ounces) kale, chard, or other dark leaves, chopped fine

3 large sheets of toasted nori (seaweed)

Salt and pepper

10 to 12 ounces salmon or herring with skin, cooked or canned, and broken into chunks

2 to 6 tablespoons fat (at least half coconut oil, but throw in some butter or ghee if you like)

3 eggs, fried, soft-boiled, or hard-boiled. Just get them in there.

IN a large soup pot over medium-high heat, bring the stock and kombu to a boil and cook for about 3 minutes. Add the leaves and boil for another 5 to 10 minutes.

REMOVE from the heat, and add the nori and season with salt and pepper. Stir to combine.

PUT the fish, fat, and eggs into a large bowl and pour the soup over it. Serve hot.

Blue cheese macadamia nut dessert

If you like blue cheese, this dish is heaven. The macadamia nuts add a delicious crunch, and every spoonful feels indulgent. SERVES 8

1 cup plain unsweetened Greek yogurt

1 cup blue cheese crumbles

1 handful or more of macadamia nuts

MIX together the yogurt, blue cheese, and macadamia nuts in a medium bowl.

POUR about ¼ cup each into dessert glasses and serve to any friends or dinner guests who like blue cheese.

Breakfast chocolate

I learned how to make this from a neat low-carb food blog called chocolatecoveredkatie.com. My recipe is different, and is more my "dump it in, mix it up, hope for the best" style. To me, this tastes better than the chocolate with 80 percent cocoa you can buy at the store—plus it has macadamia nuts in it. My wife is a chocolate wimp, but even she says this isn't bad. MAKES ABOUT 2 POUNDS

Butter, for greasing the baking dish

1½ cups of macadamia nuts or almonds (make sure there's at least one nut in every chunk, so throw in a little extra)

One (14-ounce) jar coconut oil, or 7 ounces coconut oil plus 7 ounces salted butter

3 cups (8 ounces) unsweetened cocoa powder

1 tablespoon NuStevia or other nonsugar sweetener

⅔ teaspoon salt

1½ cups shredded unsweetened coconut

Chia seeds, to taste. They actually add nothing to the taste but a little to the texture.

Raspberries (if using)

GREASE a 9-by-13-inch baking dish with butter, or use a nonstick pan. Add the nuts and spread out evenly.

HEAT the coconut oil in a double boiler over low heat until melted, or in a glass container for about 90 seconds in a microwave. Most jars of coconut oil are 14 ounces, so just take off the metal lid and heat it up in the jar.

MIX the cocoa powder, sweetener, salt, shredded coconut, and chia seeds in a large bowl. Stir to blend thoroughly with a whisk or a fork. Add the warm liquid coconut oil and stir in thoroughly. Pour the mixture over the nuts in the prepared baking dish. Make sure all the nuts are buried in the chocolate.

YOU CAN also add raspberries to it. Vary the recipe to suit, but this is a good foundation.

STICK the chocolate bark in the freezer, and it'll be ready to eat in 10 minutes. Break into chunks with a knife.

SERVE and eat it out of the refrigerator or freezer, cool to cold. On mornings when I don't feel like a real breakfast but do feel like chomping on something, I'll eat a few chunks of this. It has zero effect on my blood glucose.

OUTGROW THIS BOOK

If you've read this far, you know how food and exercise affect your body, and have enough of an understanding of the way carbohydrates and anaerobic exercise affect you to dive into any of the more comprehensive books and blogs listed below. In most cases, the authors are professionals, academics, or scholars beyond my league, and go into more detail than I do. They all agree that minimizing blood sugar and insulin is key to good health, but sometimes they disagree about fat (like, how much, what kind?), fiber (do we need any?), and fruit (are the antioxidants worth the fructose?). I list these sources to explain my influences, and to publicly thank the authors for flipping me around. If you want a deeper level of detail or simply can't get enough of this stuff, I highly recommend them all.

Books

Bowden, Jonny, PhD, CNS, and Stephen Sinatra, MD, FACC. *The Great Cholesterol Myth.* Lions Bay, BC (Canada): Fair Winds Press, 2012.

If you have a decent diet and still worry about your cholesterol numbers, this book will fix that.

Cordain, Loren, PhD. *The Paleo Diet.* New York: John Wiley & Sons, 2002.

Loren Cordain coined "paleo diet" with this book, and got the modern ball rolling.

Cunnane, Stephen C. *Survival of the Fattest: The Key to Human Brain Evolution.* Singapore: World Scientific Publishing, 2005.

Cunnane explains the importance of fat, seafood, and the nutrients the brain needs to develop.

Davis, Ellen. *Fight Cancer with a Ketogenic Diet.* ketogenic-diet-resource.com, 2013.

Ellen Davis sums up the promise of ketones in fighting cancer, and explains clearly the findings of Dr. Thomas Seyfried, a leader in the use of ketogenic diets to fight cancer. It's an ebook only.

Eades, Michael R., MD, and Mary Dan Eades, MD. *Protein Power.* New York: Bantam Books, 1996.

The title is misleading, since most of the book is pro-fat and anti-carb more than it is pro-protein. It has more information and detail not covered in other low-carb books, including this one.

——. *The 30-Day Low-Carb Diet Solution.* Hoboken, NJ: John Wiley & Sons, 2003.

Enig, Mary, PhD. *Know Your Fats: The Complete Guide for Understanding the Nutrition of Fats, Oils, and Cholesterol.* Silver Spring, MD: Bethesda Press, 2000.

Gedgaudas, Nora. *Primal Body, Primal Mind.* Rochester, VT: Healing Arts Press, 2011.

The author is a nutritional therapist who attacks hippie and right-wing nutrition with equal zeal, and explains the science behind low-carb, low-fiber, high-fat eating.

Hahn, Frederick, Michael R. Eades, MD, and Mary Dan Eades, MD. *The Slow Burn Fitness Revolution.* New York: Broadway Books, 2005.

The benefits of exercising more slowly, from the coauthors of *Protein Power.*

Keith, Lierre. *The Vegetarian Myth.* Crescent City, CA: Flashpoint Press, 2009.

The author, a former vegan, tells how she got her health back by eating meat, and the dangers of doing without it.

Kossoff, Eric H., MD, John M. Freeman, MD, Zahava Turner, RD, and James E. Rubenstein, MD. *Ketogenic Diets.* New York: Demos Medical Publishing, 2011.

Clinical information on ketogenic diets, particularly for epilepsy, but general information, too.

Lieberman, Daniel E. *The Evolution of the Human Head.* Cambridge, MA: Belknap Press/Harvard University Press, 2011.

If you're cramped for time, focus on the first few chapters, which discuss the shaping of the skull.

Mackarness, Richard, MD. *Eat Fat and Grow Slim.* London: Harvill Press, 1958.

This book predates Atkins by more than a decade, but timing is everything. If this book were published anytime after 1990, it would have sold millions of copies. The title says it all.

Monastyrsky, Konstantin. *Fiber Menace.* Lyndhurst, NJ: Ageless Press, 2008.

The author goes beyond suggesting that fiber is a harmless sham. He makes a case for its being harmful. If you're concerned about not getting enough, read any page of this book.

Moore, Jimmy, with Eric Westman, MD. *Cholesterol Clarity.* Victory Belt Publishing, 2013.

How to interpret the numbers in your cholesterol test, why they might not be cause for alarm if they're high, and how eating fat can improve them.

Newport, Mary T., MD. *Alzheimer's Disease: What If There Was a Cure?* Laguna Beach, CA: Basic Health Publications, 2013.

Dr. Newport's husband got Alzheimer's, and she arrested and slightly reversed it with coconut oil. If Alzheimer's disease is part of your life or family, you'll find hope and practical advice here.

Ruhl, Jenny. *Blood Sugar 101.* Turners Falls, MA: Technion Books, 2012.

The author is diabetic and has studied her own body as a way to get to the bottom of managing it. Every diabetic should read it.

Shaw, Judith. *Trans Fats: The Hidden Killer in Our Food.* New York: Simon & Schuster, 2004.

If you harbor any doubts about the dangers of trans-fats, this book will remove them with force.

Sisson, Mark. *The Primal Blueprint.* Malibu, CA: Primal Nutrition, 2009.

Mark is an excellent writer and researcher, enthusiastic but never goofy. His blog is must-reading for all low-carbers. marksdailyapple.com/

Stevens, C. Edward, and Ian D. Hume. *Comparative Physiology of the Vertebrate Digestive System.* Cambridge, U.K.: Cambridge University Press, 1995.

An authoritative textbook that cuts through the conflicting digestion information on the Internet.

Taubes, Gary. *Good Calories, Bad Calories.* New York: Alfred A. Knopf, 2007.

A weighty, comprehensive, fascinating guide to blood sugar, insulin, carbohydrates, and most of the problems they cause and make worse.

——. *Why We Get Fat.* New York: Alfred A. Knopf, 2011.

If you read only three books on this list, this should be one of them. It is a shorter and more accessible version of Taubes's earlier book, *Good Calories, Bad Calories,* and has helped thousands of people understand why they need to cut out carbs.

Tsatsouline, Pavel. *Enter the Kettlebell!* St. Paul, MN: Dragon Door Publications, 2006. (Also available on DVD.)

Pavel Tsatsouline introduced kettlebells in the United States, and his books and videos are helpful for anybody who wants to get strong. He is authoritative, built like an iron rope, and has a sense of humor that makes him quite likeable. Believe Pavel.

Voegtlin, Walter L. *The Stone Age Diet.* New York: Vantage Press, 1975.

This book is no longer in print, but is available online as a pdf. Find the pdf, then email it to a printer and have it spiral bound. Fascinating reading. You'll wonder why it wasn't a bestseller.

Volek, Jeff S., PhD, RD, and Stephen D. Phinney, MD, PhD. *The Art and Science of Low Carbohydrate Living.* Miami, FL: Beyond Obesity, 2011.

The authors are experts and excellent writers. Essential reading.

——. *The Art and Science of Low Carbohydrate Performance.* Miami, FL: Beyond Obesity, 2012.

If you're coming at this from a history of competition and are concerned about performance drop-offs, read this and relax.

Wade, Paul. *Convict Conditioning.* St. Paul, MN: Dragon Door Publications, 2009.

In the old days before convicts had gyms, they had to get strong in a cell with only a bunk, a toilet, and their own body weight. The author first went to jail weighing 120 pounds, and within six months became strong enough to coach the other inmates. The last word on body-weight exercise.

Westman, Eric, MD. *A Low-Carbohydrate, Ketogenic Diet Manual.* © Eric C. Westman, MD, MHS, 2013.

A 24-page manual about ketogenic diets, available online. It costs about $5.00. Just get it.

Westman, Eric C., MD, Stephen D. Phinney, MD, and Jeff S. Volek, PhD. *The New Atkins for a New You.* New York: Simon & Schuster, 2010.

This is the modern, updated version of the original Atkins diet book. Fantastic.

Wolf, Robb. *The Paleo Solution.* Victory Belt Publishing, 2010.

The author is a former student of Loren Cordain (*The Paleo Diet),* and is expert in all things related to low-carb diets and fitness.

Wrangham, Richard. *Catching Fire.* New York: Basic Books, 2009.

How eating easily digestible meat helped woodland apes evolve to become human.

Websites and blogs

Carolyn Ketchum, low-ish carb meals and desserts: alldayidreamaboutfood.com

Dana Carpenter: holdthetoast.com

Denise Minger: rawfoodsos.com

Jimmy Moore: livinlowcarbdiscussion.com

Katie, low-carb versions of traditional sweets: chocolatecoveredkatie.com

Kris Gunnars: authoritynutrition.com

Mark Sisson: marksdailyapple.com

Michael Eades, MD: proteinpower.com

Mike Evans, MD: Google "23½ hours"
In a 9-minute video, Dr. Mike does more for walking than anybody since *Homo erectus*.

National Institutes of Health: original studies on all aspects of health: NIH.com

Nutrition Science Initiative, founded by Gary Taubes and Peter Attia, to fund studies: nusi.org

Peter Attia, MD: theeatingacademy.com

Robb Wolf: robbwolf.com

INDEX

A

ab wheel, 132–133

acetoacetate, 21, 160

acetone, 21, 160, 169

advice, bad, 179, 180, 184–185

Aerobics (Cooper), 68

alcohol, 27, 55–56

Alzheimer's disease, 173–174

amaranth, 36

American Diabetes Association, 184

American push-ups, 88–89

amylase, 171–172

antibiotics, 154–155

antioxidants, 41–42, 63

appendix, 152

artery health, 164

artificial sweeteners, 58

Atkins, Robert, 19–20

Atkins diet, 19–20

Australopithecus afarensis, 144, 146

avian digestive system, 150–151, 153

avocados, 63

B

bacon grease, 32

bacteria, beneficial, 154

barley, 36

beef fat, 32

beer, 27, 55–56

bell peppers, 63

berries, 63

beta-hydroxybutyrate, 21, 160, 169

bicycles, 139

blood pressure, 51–52

blood sugar levels, 166–167, 179. ***See also*** glucose

blue cheese and cherry tomato soup, 202

blue cheese macadamia nut dessert, 205

body types, 75

body-weight exercises, description of, 87

Brazil nuts, 44–45

breakfast, 24, 34

breakfast chocolate, 206–207

broccoli, 192, 193–194

buckwheat, 36

burpees, 125–127

butter, 32

C

calories, exercise and, 72–73
cancer, 162
carbohydrates
  overview of, 4–5
  role of, 2
  in whole grains, 36–37
cardiovascular health, 184–185
cats, 183
celiac disease, 156
cellulose, 5
cereal, 36
"cereal," super white, 198
cheese, 63, 154
children, 179, 181
chocolate, 57, 206–207
chocolate mousse alternative, 199
chocoroons, 200
cholesterol, 30, 43, 163, 164
clean, squat, press, 116–119, 127
clothing, workout, 71
cocoa powder, 199, 201, 206–207
coconut, 47–48, 62, 200, 202, 206–207
coconut butter, 47, 201
coconut flakes, 198, 201
coconut milk, 47, 198, 202, 203
coconut oil, 32, 47, 62, 173–174, 206–207
coconut water, 48
complex carbohydrates, 4
Cooper, Kenneth, 68
Cordain, Loren, 20
corn, 36, 38–39, 60
corn syrup, 39, 40
correlations, 175
cortisol, 68, 75
cost estimates, 64–65
countdowns, 128, 129
crawling, 98–99
cream, fun with, 199
Crohn's disease, 156
croutons, 197

D

daily diet, 17–18
de la Monte, Suzanne, 173
diabetes, 161, 165
diabetes-safe croutons, 197
diet
  daily, 17–18
  guidelines for, 23
  low-carb, 19–21
digestive systems, 148, 149–153
dinners, low-carb, 25–26
dips, 96–97
dogs, 183
downhill sit-ups, 90–92
dynamic stretching, 84–85

E

easy days, 141
eggplant, 191, 195–196
eggs, 43, 62, 190, 192, 200, 204–205
18-hour fast, 7
energy bars, 59
erythritol, 57, 58

Eskimos, 13
evolutionary biology, 144–147
exercise
- clothing for, 71
- effective, 70
- exertion and, 82
- fun and, 80
- gyms and, 78–79
- overview of, 67
- routine for, 77
- spread it out, 141

F

fake pizza with no crust, 191
fantastic blue cheese dressing, 203
fantastic fake pancakes, 190
fantastic fake quiche, 192
fasting, 7–8
fasting blood sugar score, 166–167
fat
- bad, 30–31
- body, 1, 2, 157–158, 159–161, 178
- as friend, 1
- as fuel, 15
- good, 28–29
- heat and, 31, 32
- storage of, 33

fatty acids, 163
fecal transplants, 154
fermentation, 155
fiber, 35
Fibonacci, 131
Fibonacci pyramids, 130
fire, 146
fish, 28, 29, 61, 66, 144, 145, 204–205
Food Pyramid, 22
free weights, 78
fructose, 40, 59
fruit/fruit juice, 40, 59
fun with cream, 199

G

General Mills, 36
ghee, 32
gluconeogenesis, 68, 75, 159–160
glucose, 2, 40, 74, 157–158, 159, 165
gluten intolerance, 156
Glycemic Index (GI), 49–50
glycerol, 163
glycogen, 159
grains, 35–37, 59
Greek yogurt, 54, 154, 198, 203, 205
green soup, 193–194
growth hormone, 181
guilt, 186

H

halfway sit-ups, 92
HDL (high-density lipoprotein), 30, 164
high-fructose corn syrup, 39, 40
hills, 138, 139
homeostasis, 72, 73, 157–158
Homo erectus, 145–146

Homo habilis, 145
Homo sapiens, 147
hotel exercising, 140
hunger, 6, 12, 157–158
hydrogenated oil, 60

I

injury prevention, 95, 96
insulin
- Alzheimer's disease and, 173
- diabetes and, 161, 165
- exercise and, 72
- lowering, 1, 7–8
- role of, 2–3, 157–158
- sensitivity to, 9

J

Janda sit-ups, 90–92
Japaneasy soup, 204–205
jogging, 68–69
jumping, 102
jump-starts, 96–97

K

kangaroo jumps, 102
kefir cheese, 154
ketoacidosis, 161
ketogenesis, 160
ketogenic diet, 20–21, 162
ketones, 20–21, 47, 160, 168–170
ketosis, 19, 21, 159–161, 168
kettlebell exercises
- clean, squat, press, 116–119, 127
- description of, 87
- one-hand swing, 108
- snatch, 110–112
- squat, 109
- Turkish get-up, 113–115
- two-hand swing, 105–108, 127
- windmills, 120–122

kettlebells, 78, 103–104
killer burpees, 125–127
kimchi, 154
Koichi, Irisawa, 124
kombucha tea, 154

L

lactic acid, 76
lactose, 54, 63
lard, 32
LDL (low-density lipoprotein), 30, 163, 164
leafy greens, 5, 41–42, 61–62, 155
Leonardo of Pisa, 131
let-downs, 94–95, 96
ligaments, 84
lipoproteins, 164
low-carb foods, 10–11

M

macadamia nuts, 44, 205, 206–207
macadamia oil, 32, 62
maize, 39
maltitol, 57
maltodextrine, 58
mealtimes, 187
meat, 62

medicine ball fetch, 134–135
medium-chain triglycerides (MCTs), 29, 47, 62, 173–174
menus, sample, 65
microbiome, 154–155
millet, 36
miso soup, 154
moderation, 9
momentum, 81
momentum sit-ups, 92
monogastric carnivores, 151–152
monogastric digestive system, 151–152, 153
monogastric herbivores, 152
monogastric omnivores, 152
monounsaturated fats, 28–29, 46
mushrooms, 63
MyPlate, 22

N

negative pull-ups, 94–95
90 percent fat fast, 7–8
no-carb foods, 10
nori, 204–205
Normann, Wilhelm, 30
NuStevia, 58
Nutrition Science Initiative, 176
nuts, 44–45

O

oats, 36
oils, 28–29, 30–31
olive oil, 32, 33, 46, 62
omega-3 fatty acids, 28–29, 61
omega-6 fatty acids, 28–29, 31, 43, 44
omnivores, 156
on-and-offs, 139
one-hand swing, 108
organ meats, 62

P

Paleo diet, 20
pancakes, fantastic fake, 190
pancreas, 165
partially hydrogenated oil, 60
peppers, 63
PET (positron emission tomography) scan, 162
pets, 183
phytic acid, 53
phytoestrogens, 53
phytonutrients, 41–42
pickles, 154
Pisano, Leonardo, 131
pizza, fake with no crust, 191
potassium, 63
potatoes, 49–50, 59
prebiotics, 154–155
press, 118–119
Primal Blueprint Diet, 20
probiotics, 154
protein, 14, 37
pseudoruminants, 150, 153
pull-ups, 94–95
push-ups, 88–89, 93, 126–127

Q

quiche, fantastic fake, 192
quinoa, 37

R

raised torso sit-ups, 92
real ratatouille, 195–196
recipes, overview of, 189
refined carbohydrates, 4
repetitive countdowns, 129
reps, 76, 81
resources, 209–216
rice, 36, 37, 60
ruminants, 149–150, 153
Russian push-ups, 88–89
rye, 37

S

salmon, 61, 204–205
salt, 51
sandwiches, breadless, 16
sauerkraut, 154
scientific studies, 175–176
seed oils, 30–31
selenium, 44–45
Sisson, Mark, 20
sitting, 83
sit-ups, 90–92
smoke points, 32
snatch, kettlebell, 110–112
soybeans, 53
spinach, 192
sports drinks, 59
sprinting, 136–137
squats, 100–101, 109, 118
squat-thrusts, 125–127
stair climbing, 140
standing workstations, 83
static stretching, 84
Stefansson, Vilhjalmur, 13
stevia, 48, 57, 58
stretching, 84–85
sugars, 59, 162
  fake, 58
sumo wrestlers, 17
super white "cereal," 198
supplements, 13, 31
swimming, 140

T

Tabata, Izumi, 123, 124
Tabatas, 79, 123–124
taste, recalibrating, 182
teenagers, 181
teosinte, 38
tomatoes, 195–196, 202
trans fats, 30, 60
triglycerides, 40, 157–158, 159–160, 163, 164
triticale, 37
Truvia, 48
Tsatsouline, Pavel, 103
Turkish get-up, 113–115
two-hand swing, 105–108, 127

V

variety, 10–11
vegetables, 41–42

W

walking, 82
warm-ups, for sprints, 136–137
warming down, 86
weight machines, 78
weight training, 76
wheat, whole, 37
windmills, 120–122
wine, 27, 55–56

Y

yogurt, Greek, 54, 154, 198, 203, 205
yolks, 43

Z

zucchini, 193–194, 195–196